FOR THE LOVE OF OPIUM

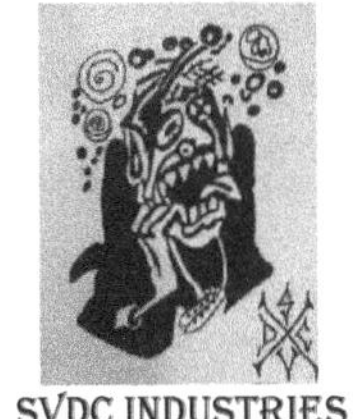

SVDC INDUSTRIES

FOR THE LOVE OF OPIUM

NATURE'S MOST POWERFUL MEDICINE

By W. E. Simmons

Published by
SVDC InDUSTries
An imprint of California Sober™
P.O. Box 181
Venice, California 90294
TheSVDC.com

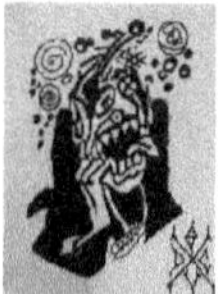

To those who loved her first

We all share in your pain

To those who left too soon

Your memories remain

To those who've yet to taste

Keep pure of mind and soul

For if you don't, you'll surely chase

Yet never fill the hole

This book is dedicated to the many we have lost.

SVDC

Us, We Rule

INTRODUCTION
FROM HEAVEN TO HELL ON EARTH

There were opium dens where one could buy oblivion, dens of horror where the memory of old sins could be destroyed by the madness of sins that were new.

- Oscar Wilde, The Picture of Dorian Gray (1891).

The century-old quote conjures an image of a darkened room in which the lost use their souls as fare to enter the dreamworld. A world where they can forget the unbearable horrors that are their broken lives. In this dingy basement, where shadows from alcohol lamps broadcast the silhouettes of harlots selling their wares on fluttering walls made of bedsheets, hopheads shamelessly drool on straw mats, their unlaundered shirts riddled with shadows that no light could consume, one hand barely clutching their favorite Opium pipe. Sordid malefactors leaning in shadowy corners plot to pilfer the oblivious as they nod deeply into paradise. A paradise so sublime that their only thoughts upon waking are of how to scam another hit.

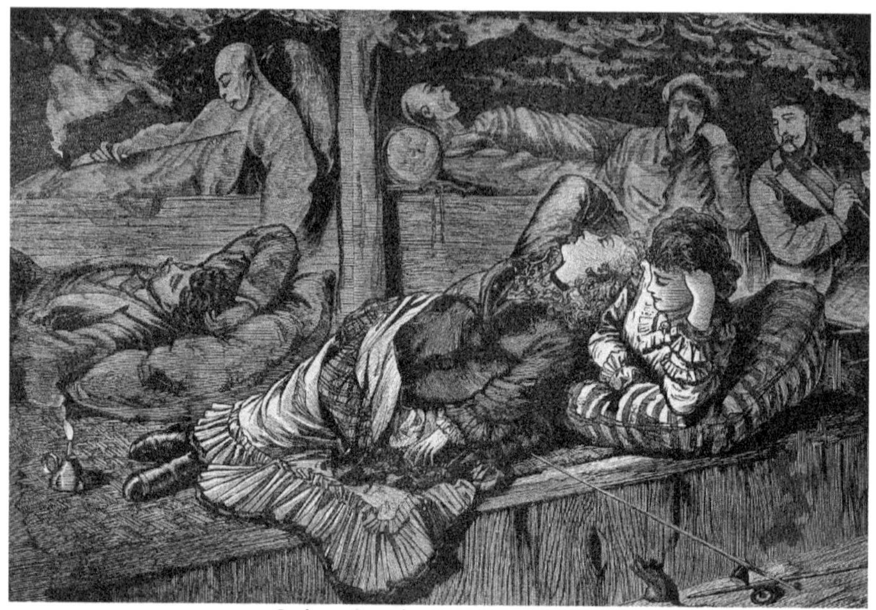

Opium Den in San Francisco.
Image published in Finnish periodical Suomen Kuvalehti, 29 February 1876

That image bears a striking resemblance to the life of an opiate lover today, save for some key distinctions. The dens are now street corners and abandoned buildings where women and men are willing to trade sexual favors to strangers, ones they would otherwise find repulsive and vile, in order to feed an unsatiable hunger that once began as a simple desire. A desire to feel not the pains of existence. A longing to escape the torturous lives into which they were born. A yearning to feel the pleasures of the flesh. A need to feel happiness once again, if only for a moment. We can all understand the desire, we simply can't fathom what it would take to abandon our lives in search of it.

Instead of a pipe, they loosely clutch their needle. That is if it isn't still sticking out of their arm like a tranquilizer dart protruding from the flesh of a wild animal. Passed-out junkies are robbed of their drugs, money, and possessions by the *friends* they walked in with, and would do the same in return if it meant getting a taste of the feeling they long for. Their *desire* has quietly mutated, like a cancer, into an all-consuming necessity. What was once recreation is now but daily maintenance. The poison that robs them of their health is the only medicine that can save them from the sickness. Oscar Wilde could have never imagined the horrors that the evolution of modern medicine, and its betrayal in the name of capitalism, would deliver.

The synthetic Demons they now crave have long since dominated and devoured their naturally occurring Angelic predecessors. Where Opium was the muse of Romanticism at the end of the 18th century, stronger pharmaceutical synthetics, like Fentanyl and Oxycontin, are the Sirens of destruction that consume millions of lives on an annual basis. Many argue that this is the result of government regulations and greed that lead to the cultural erasure of both herbal medicines, which all opiate painkillers are derived from, and of ritualistic and recreational use of natural compounds like those found in Papaver Somniferum, the Opium poppy. Opium, as well as countless other psychoactive plants and fungi, has been used by our ancestors since before homo sapiens ever evolved, yet has only been a crime since your grandma was a kid, but we'll get into that later.

While Oscar Wilde's Opium Den may have been the scourge of polite society, the nectar of the Gods was certainly enjoyed in high society for as long as society has existed. The Greeks, Romans, and Egyptians all enjoyed the blood of the Poppy, both medicinally and recreationally, in hospitals and at festivals. It wasn't until Opium's replacement by pharmaceuticals, the first ever being Opium's *active ingredient* - Morphine, that our love for this plant gave way to higher highs from which we may never come down. But before there were junkies, there was romance.

CHAPTER 1

MONSTERS, MAIDENS, AND MADMEN

OPIUM IN POLITE SOCIETY

From Rome to Egypt

Marcus Aurelius ruled over the great Roman Empire from 161 to 180, under the influence of Opium every day of it.[1] Whether or not he (or anyone in the Ancient World) was addicted to Opium is the subject of debate among scholars.[2] Some historians credit (or blame) his compassion, even for his enemies, to this medicine in his daily regimen. A compassion that in Marcus' time could have been seen as a sign of weakness. Others say that his Stoic philosophy was a result of his use of Opium and that it may have helped inspire his famous writings, known now as *Meditations*, considered some of the greatest works of philosophy. For Marcus, the latex of the Papaver Somniferum brought about introspection that reinforced his empathy in a time when rulers were respected for their cruelty.

Long before Marcus, Julius Caesar ruled the kingdom and famously had an extramarital affair with Cleopatra, whom he helped gain the throne of Egypt. His general Marcus Antonius, or Mark Antony, is also famous for his love of the Egyptian queen. Their story tragically ends when Mark Antony, mistakenly believing that his lover is dead, thrusts his sword into his stomach.

After learning Cleopatra was in fact not dead, he had himself carried to her. Soon after Marc Antony died in her arms, Cleopatra also took her own life.

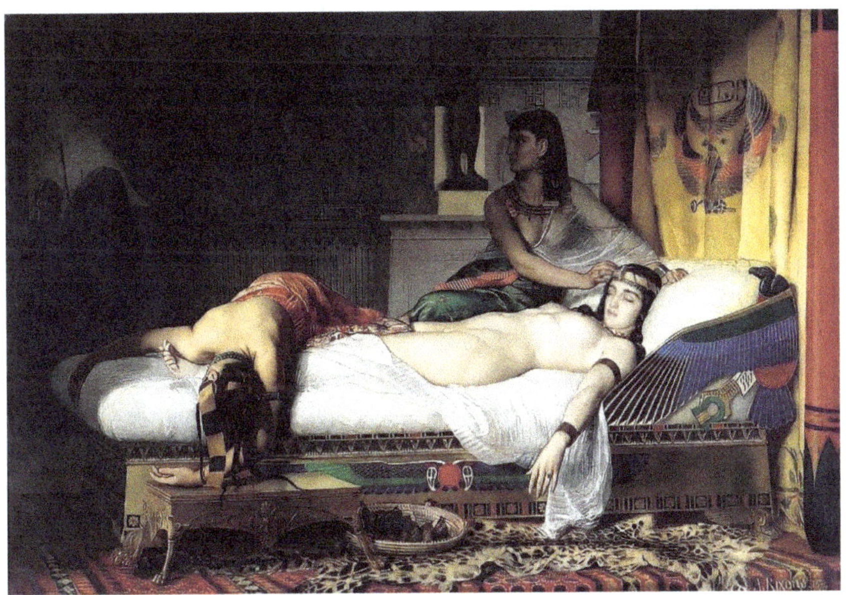

The Death of Cleopatra (1874)
By Jean-André Rixens

While for millennia legend had it that she died from the bite of a poisonous snake that she had smuggled into her chamber, the fact is that she died from an overdose of Opium,[3] along with her two handmaidens Charmion and Iras. Opium was a product that was readily available to the Queen. She had undoubtedly taken it before and knew of its calming nature and psychotropic pleasures. She also knew that it would cause an easy death, as she had already researched the best ways to die. Cleopatra administered different poisons to her prisoners while watching their effects unfold. She studied death, knowing one day she would likely have to cause her own, finding the juice of the Poppy to be the most peaceful manner.

Romantics, Writers, Actors and Poets

Edgar Allan Poe also used Opium, in the form of Laudanum, possibly as an attempt on his own life. Perhaps, one might speculate, it was simply a dramatic way to gain the attention of the woman he loved. He figured that if he was at death's door the woman he desired, Annie Richmond, would run to his side. He purchased two ounces of Laudanum and wrote her a letter informing her of his plan to commit suicide. He took about half of the Opium cocktail before leaving to mail the letter, planning to take the other half upon Annie's arrival. Before he reached the post office he was doped up and out of his mind. He completely forgot where he was going, and for what reason. A *friend,* Poe later confessed, *was at hand* and saved him. He puked up the Laudanum and it was days before he could recall what actually happened. [4]

But sinister applications of Opium are much less common than its use for unbridled creativity. The juice of the Poppy was the catalyst of inspiration for such famous Opium users as Charles Dickens when he wrote A Christmas Carol and Oliver Twist, and his knowledge of Opium dens is outlined in detail in his final work. One can only imagine the Opium fueled dreams that led to the three ghosts that haunted Ebenezer Scrooge as he tried to catch a nod.

Samuel Taylor Coleridge, writer of The Rime of the Ancient Mariner, used Opium to quiet his anxiety and possible bipolar disorder. He wrote Kubla Kahn, among other notable works, while under the influence of this powerful elixir. He kept his use mostly secret until his pal, Thomas De Quincy, ratted him out to the world in his famous manuscript *Confessions of an English Opium-Eater*.

Actor Bella Lugosi was infamous for his addiction to Opiates. He was said to frequent underground Opium dens while creating the screen's first Dracula, a work so eerily convincing that critics questioned whether or not the actor was truly a vampire. And that vampire may have never been played had it not been for an Opium and alcohol-fueled summer, according to the accounts of authors Mary Shelly and John Polidori.

Sex, Drugs, and Monsters - Frankenstein and The Vampyre

The story of our most beloved monsters begins when a young poet and avid Opium enthusiast Percy Shelley sought out the mentorship of his idol William Godwin, author of *Political Justice*. Percy was infatuated with the Anarchist, as well as the work of Godwin's late wife, Mary Wollstonecraft, the inspiration for Shelley's *free love* philosophy. At least partially due to their influence, Percy himself became anti-government, anti-religion (he was a devout atheist), and anti-monogamy. He promoted the idea that one should be free to have sex with whomever they felt love for without the burdens of guilt, jealousy, and commitment.

Shelley began correspondence with Godwin in an attempt to obtain his mentorship, going so far as to ask if Mary Wollstonecraft's illegitimate daughter, Fanny Imlay, could come live with him and his wife, Harriet Westbrook. Godwin smartly refused but continued writing Shelley in the hopes that his protégé would help him with his financial troubles. Percy eventually began visiting the Godwin family almost daily in May of 1814.

Percy was an accomplished cocksman, adept at seduction. His infatuation with his then-wife, Harriet Westbrook, began when he was mourning the end of a romantic relationship with his cousin, Harriet Grove. During his 5-year marriage to Miss Westbrook, Shelley became infatuated with an unmarried schoolteacher named Elizabeth Hitchener and even asked her to come live with him and his new wife. Early in 1814, he fell for a woman by the name of Cornelia Turner (and also her mother, Harriet de Boinville). By April of that year, he turned his love to Frances (Fanny) Imlay.

In such a chaste society, Percy must have been quite a wordsmith to seduce so many women, even attempting to move some of them into the home he shared with his wife. One can only imagine that his hunt for sister wives wasn't limited to Elizabeth, Cornelia,

Harriet, and Fanny. It should have been little surprise that Percy seduced all three of the young women of the Godwin house, Fanny Imlay, Mary Godwin, and Claire Clairmont, William Godwin's stepdaughter.

Mary and Percy began meeting at her mother's grave where Mary eventually gave Percy her virginity. Interestingly, Mary was always accompanied on these rendezvous by Claire, even on the day that they consummated their relationship. Mary, who admittedly had an "excessive and romantic attachment" to her father, saw Percy as the incarnation of both her parents' beliefs. It wasn't, therefore, hard for him to conjure her attention. When Percy declared his love for the 16-year-old Mary Godwin to his then-wife Harriet, she begged the Godwins not to let him visit their home anymore. Mr. Godwin wrote to Percy, banning him from ever visiting. That lasted about a week.

Percy returned and, according to Mary's stepmother, "*He looked extremely wild. He pushed me aside with extreme violence, and entering, walked straight to Mary. 'They wish to separate us, my beloved; but Death shall unite us,' and offered her a bottle of laudanum. 'By this you can escape from tyranny; and this,' taking a small pistol from his pocket, 'shall reunite me to you.' Poor Mary turned as pale as a ghost, and my poor silly Claire, who is so timid even at trifles, at the sight of the pistol filled the room with her shrieks.*"[5]

Mary calmed him down, telling him that if he were to leave the house that very moment, she would love him forever. While he honored her wishes, their separation drove him mad. After just a week without her by his side, Percy *took a violent dose* of Laudanum. Like Poe, we can only wonder if it was actually an attempt to commit suicide, or just a dramatic attempt to regain Mary's attention. Maybe he just wanted to get really high. In any case, it served two of these purposes.

Percy and Mary, along with her stepsister Claire, ran away and traveled across Europe in an apparent free-love threesome leaving

Fanny, who had been sent to Whales by her father in order to be far from Percy, behind. It was rumored that Mr. Godwin sold the girls to Percy, but that was undoubtedly not the case considering that Godwin was so mad at Mary that he refused to speak with her. The three spent their downtime reading books by Mary's late mother and keeping a joint journal of their adventures that were documented in Mary Shelley's diaries and in her and Percy's travel narrative *History of a Six Weeks' Tour* (1817).

The throuple traveled through war-torn France, reading, writing, and consuming Opium and wine, eventually ending up in Switzerland where Claire would meet up with her other lover, a famous English poet by the name of Lord Byron. Mary, Percy, and Claire settled in and enjoyed Geneva for just over a week before they were joined by Byron, from whom Clair was secretly pregnant, and his personal physician and writer John William Polidori.

After some fun in the sun, boating on Lake Geneva, and sightseeing, the weather quickly changed. Dismal rain left the five indoors for most of their time there. Mary would later write about the year without a summer, saying *incessant rain often confined us for days to the house*. By that fate, the group read, wrote, and discussed politics and the supernatural while drinking copious amounts of alcohol and Laudanum. One can only imagine, based on what we now know of this free-loving threesome, what else these Opium crazed intellectuals were up to.

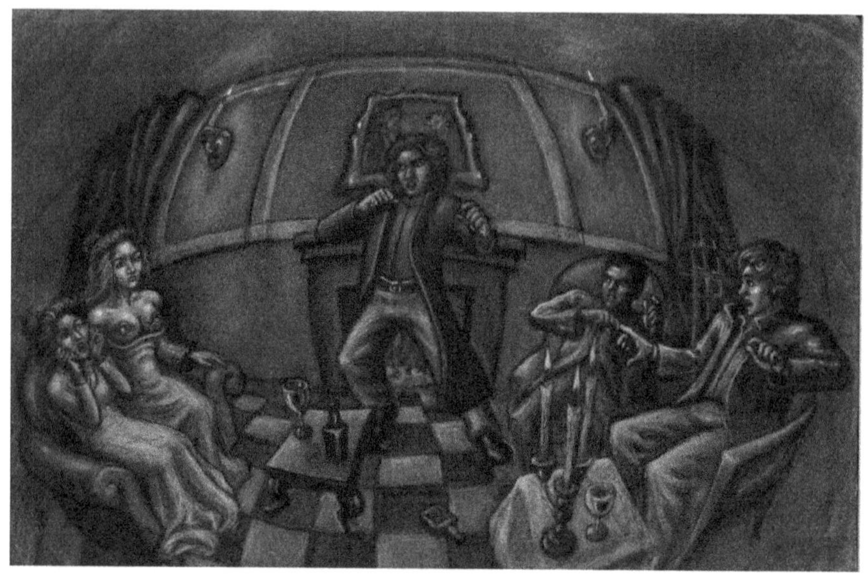

Opium, Monsters, and Madness
Andrew Z. Gardner

One evening, during a fun-filled night of alcohol and Opium fueled madness, the group took turns reading from a French anthology of German ghost stories entitled *Fantasmagoriana*. Hallucinating that Mary's nipples had turned into demonic eyes, Percy Shelley ran shrieking from the room.[6] One might assume, based on Percy's hallucinations, that they may have had better party favors than simply opiates. Soon after, Byron proposed the group each write their own individual *ghost stories.* The anxiety of the task left Mary Shelley dreading the question asked of her each morning, *have you thought of a story?*

The result of the contest was not what any of them might have imagined. Percy and Lord Byron, already published authors, lost the game, writing no ghost stories while on that vacation. Still, Byron's challenge, and quite a bit of Opium, inspired Mary Shelley to write a short story about a fictional young scientist from the most distinguished family of Geneva, where the story was written. Her protagonist, Victor, pursues the sciences due to his early interests in alchemy, specifically alchemists such as Paracelsus (the original inventor of Laudanum). He comes to assemble a humanoid creature from the parts of different corpses and brings it to life with electricity. Mary Shelley's tale of corpse reanimation would eventually become one of the most well-known horror stories of all time. Frankenstein; or, The Modern Prometheus.

In that same writing session, John Polidori wrote *The Vampyre*, which gave rise to the Vampire genre we know today. Before that work, stories of vampires were folklore and poetry depicting grotesque creatures inhabiting the underbelly of society. Not only did Polidori write the first vampire novel and start the genre we know today, but he was also the first to create a vampire who was a Nobleman with all the charm and riches of the polite society they themselves were a part of. Without that night, there may have been no Dracula for our friend Bella Lugosi to play. If it hadn't been for that summer of sex, Opium, and ghost stories in 1816, the two most iconic monster tales of all time may never have seen the darkness of night.

While the ins and outs of the group, pun intended, are stories one could write a novel about, this story is about Opium. That said, the group's love story ends with all the dread and horrors of the genre they helped make great. Not long after Opium helped to inspire those haunting creatures, Fanny Imlay took her own life with Laudanum and Percy's wife drowned herself, both the result of their love for Shelley and his devotion to Mary Godwin. Shelly went on to take several lovers on the side before his death in a boating accident. When his body was cremated on the beach, his heart refused to burn.

29 years later, when Mary Shelly passed, their only living son found his father's heart in a box on her desk, wrapped in a piece of silk that also held a bit of his ashes and a torn-out passage from Percy's poem Adonais. Mary Shelly had kept the promise that she made that evening that Percy busted into her father's house with a pistol and a bottle of Opium tincture. She swore that she would love him forever, and she kept her promise.

Other Artists

Lord Byron's daughter, Ada Lovelace, is widely referred to as the world's first computer programmer due to her work with inventor Charles Babbage on his idea for an *analytical engine* in the 1800s. She was prescribed laudanum, to be taken with wine, by her doctor. Like her father, who was said to sip laudanum out of a crystal decanter, she was an Opium user until she left this world due to cancer when she was 36. She was also friends with Charles Dickens, mentioned previously, whom she asked to visit her in the end so that he may read to her an account of death from one of his books.

Even Pablo Picasso and his close circle of friends enjoyed Opium nights at Le Bateau-Lavoir. In his studio, the 24-year-old artist and his girlfriend, Fernande Olivier, could be found, along with whomever else in the building that wished to partake, laying on straw mats, passing around a bowl of opium, and smoking out of his favorite bamboo pipe. He smoked several times a week from 1904 to 1908. The party ended when his friend, Karl-Heinz Wiegels, killed himself when he suffered a psychotic break after a night of opium, hashish, and ether. I'd estimate that the ether had more to do with his *break* than either of the others.

One of Picasso's works, *Opium Smoker with Woman in Slippers on her Bed, and a Little Dog,* from Pablo Picasso's largest print series *347 Suite*, depicts a man smoking Opium from a pipe at the foot of a woman's bed. The woman is nude, other than slippers, and her vagina and anus are predominantly displayed, possibly alluding to Opium's aphrodisiacal qualities. Most of the 347 works from that collection, as graphic as they are, show that the 87-year-old artist never lost his love of female anatomy. Its creation 60 years after the artist allegedly quit smoking Opium goes to show that his love for her also never truly ceased.

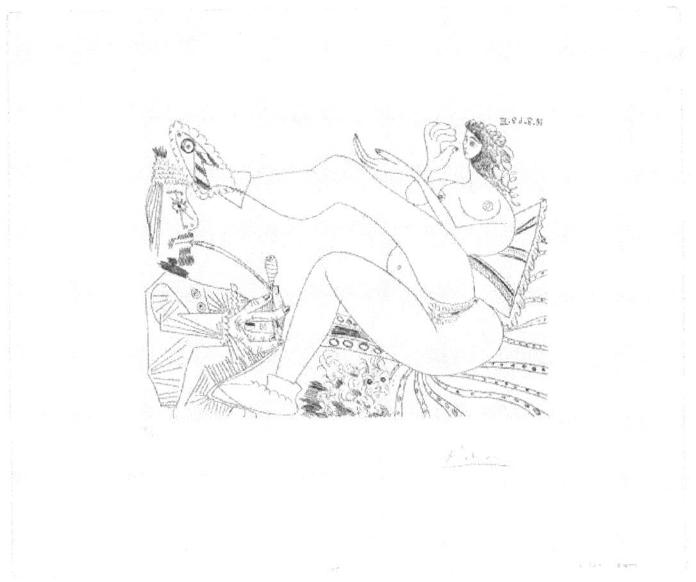

Opium Smoker with Woman in Slippers on her Bed and a Little Dog, from 347 Suite
© 2023 Estate of Pablo Picasso / Artists Rights Society (ARS), New York

Other famous users include poet and Opium enthusiast Jean Cocteau (*Opium - Diary of a Cure*), Hector Berlioz, Elizabeth Barrett Browning (*How Do I love thee? Let me count the Ways* and *Opium-opium-night after night*), and John Keats, to name just a few. Early screen Actor Errol Flynn wrote of his time frequenting Opium dens with a Eurasian hooker and scam artist named Ting Ling in his autobiography *My Wicked, Wicked Ways*.

A young Winston Churchill chewed Cocaine gum and drank Laudanum with the youthful Queen Victoria. Florence Nightingale, arguably the most famous nurse who ever walked the earth, was also hitting the stash. It wasn't hard, in her line of work, to get a free high. She has been quoted as saying "*I could not have got through the day without this wonderful little pick-me-up.*" She enjoyed that little pick-me-up for 40 years after her first Opium injection.

Opium - As American as Apple Pie

Opium was a part of the New World from the very beginning and aided in its foundation. Deacon Samuel Fuller carried Opium with him on the Mayflower, thus becoming the first physician to enter the New World. He used it to treat a later group led by John Endicott, the founder of Salem, and an even later group in Charlestown. Upon his death, 13 years after his arrival, he was praised as a surgeon, physician, and godly man. I'm sure his Opium helped him in all those endeavors.

The founding fathers of the United States also loved the Poppy's medicine. George Washington, the first president of the United States of America, famously had wooden dentures, right? As popular as the tale is, his dentures were made from real teeth, both of cows and his lone surviving natural tooth. Later, he had a set made from ivory that was carved out of hippopotamus tusks. They fit like shit and caused him a lot of pain. No angel and no prude, Washington grew weed and, after his two-term presidency, opened a whiskey distillery on his Mount Vernon estate. He also took laudanum throughout his presidency and until he died at the ripe old age of 67.

Thomas Jefferson, our third president, was skeptical of medicine as it was practiced in his time. A smart man, as they didn't really know shit about medicine in the late 1700s and early the next century, he believed in letting nature heal the body. He was an early advocate of the smallpox vaccine, not so much a medicine as a natural remedy, having his daughters and grandchildren inoculated. He suffered from headaches that his usual go-to, Peruvian bark (quinine), had begun to fail to treat. He found a cure and wrote to a friend "With care and laudanum I may consider myself to be in what is to be my habitual state." From then on, he grew his own Poppies on his Monticello estate. He used Opium until the day before his death, at which time he refused all medical treatment in order to be lucid. Papaver Somniferum was grown on that same estate until the 1990s when they were uprooted at the demand of the Drug Enforcement Administration. The government that he helped to create was no longer in favor of its founders' ideals and legacy.

Alexander Hamilton, in a letter to his wife Elizabeth on August 12, 1794, prescribed laudanum for his sick son John Church Hamilton, even telling her how to wean him off it when the time came. The first secretary of the treasury appointed by George Washington, Hamilton didn't like the third president's running mate and spoke out against his career. After six years of Hamilton disparaging Burr, Burr challenged him to an *affair of honor*, also known as a duel. They met at the site where another of Hamilton's sons, Phillip, had died in another duel while defending his father's honor. According to one account Hamilton, who had been in several *affairs of honor* that he managed to settle before a shot was fired, decided that dueling was morally wrong and shot his pistol into the air. Burr seized the opportunity and shot Hamilton through the belly and into his spine. Hamilton died the next day yet used Opium to comfort him in the meantime.

Benjamin Franklin, yet another founding father, was also an Opium user. He took Laudanum for a bladder stone that caused him terrible suffering. He continued its use for 8 years until his death at age 84. President Abraham Lincoln's wife, Mary Todd Lincoln, was also a well-known Laudanum drinker. She even attempted to buy enough to kill herself a decade after her husband's murder. Luckily for her, that sale never transpired.

CHAPTER 2

NATURE, SCIENCE, AND SYMBIOSIS

So, what is Opium, exactly?

To cure the soul by means of the senses, and the senses by means of the soul. - Oscar Wilde

The Latin word Opium comes from the Greek word opos, meaning plant juice. Opium simply means Poppy juice, specifically the juice of Papaver Somniferum or Opium Poppy. Merriam-Webster defines Opium as "a bitter brownish addictive narcotic drug that consists of the dried latex obtained from immature seed capsules of the opium poppy." The Encyclopedia Britannica says that Opium is a "narcotic drug that is obtained from the unripe seedpods of the opium poppy (Papaver Somniferum), a plant of the family Papaveraceae."

While both are technically correct, Opium is better defined as a liquid fix-all. It's no wonder it has been prescribed for anything from menstrual cramps and headaches to melancholy and unruly children. (DO NOT give it to unruly children!) She provides relief for whatever ails you, be it physical, emotional, spiritual, or otherwise. If you have bodily pain, Opium relieves it. Sadness? Opium cures that too. Bored? Not with Opium! It's hard to be angry at someone you love while under the influence so, in that way, it can even cure an argument, if both parties are willing. Anxiety is never an issue under the influence of this natural elixir, and she even contains an anticancer alkaloid.

The juice of this poppy can motivate the worst procrastinator. Opium users claim that even the most menial of tasks are easy to get through while under her spell. The one thing you would think would knock you on your ass is the same thing that'll get you off the couch and productive. Opium has been curing writer's block since the dawn of literacy. I've stared at a blank page for hours, distracting myself with anything I could find. A bit of Opium and I'm beating the keyboard faster than Dave Lombardo beats drums.

She is a gift of nature without which the world would experience immense suffering and pain, and because of which the world experiences immense suffering and pain. Opium is the likely answer to the problem yet may also be the cause. As wonderful as she is, nothing is perfect. This is partly due to the exploitation of her natural wonders, in the name of greed and profit.

The Entourage Effect Part 1

As with every natural remedy, man's natural curiosity beckons him to experiment in the hopes of finding out what makes it tick. He isolates compounds and tests their role in that plant's medicinal properties. Human intellect, blurred by our tendency for narcissism, causes us to think we have found a definitive answer, never realizing we have found but a piece of the puzzle. While we isolate alkaloids and experiment with them until we find their specific roles, we rarely question whether the entirety of the substance we started with may be in its current formula for a reason. Each of the Opium alkaloids we have discovered, along with ones we have yet to discover, may likely work best in the combination that nature delivers them.

A prime example of this is Cannabis. THC was first isolated by a Bulgarian chemist by the name of Raphael Mechoulam in 1964, yet its role in the high that Cannabis causes had been known since the 1940s. Since then, THC has been thought to be the only reason you get high. That is, until Cannabis prohibition was lifted in several states allowing for more scientific research. THC is to Cannabis as Morphine is to Opium. The reason that different strains of weed cause different effects is now known to be caused by what is called the *entourage effect*.

Cannabis Indica may cause a downer effect while Cannabis Sativa can cause a more productive and energetic high. Both get you stoned but in slightly different ways. That's because THC interacts with CBD, along with other compounds such as terpenes and flavonoids, to make a cocktail with dramatically different effects than any of its isolated alkaloids. The same is true of Opium and its natural compounds, though less research has been done on the subject.

In the same way that our bodies produce at least 20 different Endorphins, Opium produces at least 38 alkaloids, each with their own function in *our* bodies. Humans have yet to figure out which receptors to turn on and off, in cases of psychological disorders. Maybe this is because they focus on one at a time. The mind is a combination lock. You can't push one button and hope for success. The human body creates an array of chemicals to activate and deactivate switches in combinations that elude us to this day. Nature's keys can activate combinations in the mind that we don't normally use. Instead of seeing this as the superpower it is, society sees anything that makes us feel better than we normally would as trashy and sinful.

What man knows about the ways of nature is but a drop in an endless sea of ignorance. As smart as we are and as much as we have learned, we are not even close to understanding the planet we live on and the symbiosis of all living things. Again, narcissism, combined with ignorance, creates a stall in discovery. One doesn't look for the answer if he thinks he already knows it.

The cocktail, Opium, contains sugars, proteins, latex, ammonia, fats, plant wax, sulfuric and lactic acids, and a fuck ton of alkaloids. There are even Opium alkaloids that we assume have no effect because we see no result when they are used in isolation from their constituents. Opium also contains Meconic Acid, which has erroneously been called a mild narcotic. While it may not be, it may play a role in the *entourage effect,* as it binds to all the other alkaloids. Because of this bonding, screening for Meconic Acid has been used as a test to detect natural opiates.

Alkaloids

But what is an alkaloid? Well, that's what makes it all worth the work. An Alkaloid is a bitter-tasting basic organic compound, naturally occurring, that contains at least one nitrogen atom. They contain, at the very least, carbon, nitrogen, and hydrogen. Sometimes they have oxygen and/or sulfur and, more rarely, bromine, chlorine, and phosphorus. Alkaloids are, most often, either poison or pleasure. They either kill you, or they get you high.

The juice of the poppy is poisonous in large doses, yet it is not nearly as deadly as its isolated alkaloids or their synthetic counterparts. According to the Centers for Disease Control, synthetic Opioids cause tens of thousands of deaths every year, more than three times as many deaths as the compounds isolated from Opium, such as Morphine. When was the last time you heard of someone overdosing on Opium? Still, like all medicines natural and otherwise, caution should be taken when consuming any mind and body-altering substance.

Papaver Somniferum latex has a narcotic, soporific, analgesic, and astringent effect. In layman's terms, she numbs, makes you sleepy, and relieves pain. Opium contains the naturally occurring organic compounds Morphine, Codeine, Noscapine, Papaverine, and Thebaine, along with almost 40 other alkaloids in precise ratios. Possibly nature's best recipe, some alkaloids relieve a multitude of symptoms while others relieve the side effects that other alkaloids may cause. While some of the effects are similar and overlapping, each of these alkaloids has its own medicinal use and function in the body.

Morphine

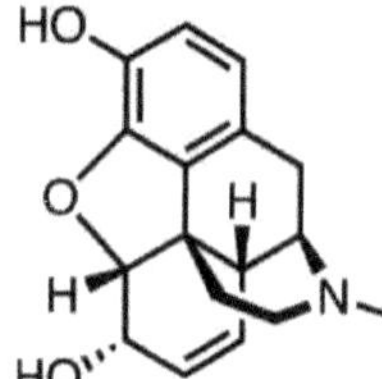

Morphine, originally called *Morphium*, was the first active alkaloid to ever be isolated from a plant, in 1804. German pharmacist Friedrich Serturner discovered Morphine when he was just 21 years old. He tried a pinch of his new find for a toothache. When he woke up several hours later, he decided that his discovery was safe for human consumption. He then began to test his new friend on himself, three young boys, a few dogs, and a mouse. While they all nearly died, he eventually figured out the dosage, the same dosage that is recommended today. He found that one *dose* of a half grain (about 30mg) induced a light and happy sensation, a second dose caused drowsiness, and a third made the volunteers confused and somnolent. He decided that the best dose was a conservative 15mg. Even now, the recommended dose of Morphine starts at 15-30mg. Not long after his discovery, he became a recluse and used Morphine regularly until his death at age 57 (not from Morphine, by the way).

Morphine is also an endogenous opioid in humans, meaning that it is synthesized and released from many different cells in our bodies, including white blood cells. Our own immune system, which is marvelous in its own right, acts almost as a separate entity in defending our bodies from invaders and helping to cure what ails us. Think of white blood cells as the body's doctors. They fight off pathogens, immobilize injuries, and make their own Morphine to help with the pain. If the manufacture of Morphine for personal use is illegal, we are all guilty as sin.

Friedrich named his find after the Greco-Roman God Morpheus, one of three sons of the god of sleep, Hypnos, Latin Somnus. Morpheus was responsible for delivering human shapes to the minds of the dreamers, while his brothers sent animal shapes and inanimate objects. In my dreams, Morpheus seems to be the hardest worker of the trio. Fittingly, Morphine is the hardest worker of all the alkaloids in Opium. It produces the strongest and most desirable effect while maintaining the highest percentage in the mixture. It acts directly on the central nervous system to induce analgesia, the inability to feel pain. When eaten, it hits in about an hour and the effects can last for 4 to 6.

A close friend of mine named Victor, known on the streets as Greasy, once told me that sleep was the cousin of death. He meant that if one sleeps all the time, he may as well be dead. Mythologically speaking, he wasn't far off. Hypnos, the Greco-Roman God of Sleep, is the twin brother of Thanatos, the God of Death. Both were sons of Nyx (night), who was the daughter of Chaos. Interesting lineage considering the close relationship between the two in Morphine.

Codeine

Codeine, the most widely used alkaloid on the planet, was discovered by the French chemist Pierre Jean Robiquet while he was attempting to refine Morphine. A brilliant man, Pierre also isolated Caffeine and discovered the first amino acid, asparagine. Yet of all his work, and for good reason, Codeine is his most famous discovery. Like Morphine, Codeine is also an endogenous opioid in humans.

Named for the Greek word for Poppy head, the source of opium, Codeine is the second most powerful naturally occurring opiate. It shares the pain-relieving and sleep-inducing properties of its cousin Morphine yet has powers all its own. While boasting exceptional pain relief and mood elevation, it also suppresses cough and relieves diarrhea. Isolated from Opium, it causes a prickly feeling on the skin and severe itching in high doses. Since I discovered it in junior high in 1984, thanks to my close friend Phantom, I loved Codeine until my arms were raw from scratching. Orally, as with most natural opiates, it hits in under an hour and lasts around 4 to 6 hours.

Noscapine

Noscapine, another find by our friend Pierre Jean Robiquet, was originally called Narcotine. He spent 20 years trying to find the best way to isolate Morphine. It's no wonder that his work with Opium would gift him yet another useful alkaloid. Its name is a variant of the word gnoscopine - from the Latin *gnos* (know) and *Op(ium)* and *ine* (of), Noscapine translates to *know of opium*, and that's what we are all trying to do here, right? Noscapine is an antitussive, or cough suppressant. Her effects are similar to dextromethorphan and alcohol intoxication and set in in about an hour or two. The almost drunk feeling of Opium is caused by a combination of these opioids. This particular alkaloid is also an anti-mitotic, a type of drug that blocks cell growth by stopping mitosis (cell division) and can be used to treat cancer. Opium truly is nature's best medicine.

Papaverine

Papaverine, whose name simply means *belonging to Papaver* (the Opium poppy), was discovered by Georg Merck in 1848. It has a wide range of recreational and pharmacological uses.

Papaverine is an antispasmodic, used to treat spasms of the gastrointestinal tract, bile ducts, and ureter. It's also used as a cerebral and coronary vasodilator in subarachnoid hemorrhage and coronary artery bypass surgery. Papaverine is used as a smooth muscle relaxant in microsurgery, where it's applied directly to blood vessels. It's also used as an erectile dysfunction medication, both topically and by injection. Shot into the base of the penis, it causes an erection. As they say, whatever floats your boat. Papaverine is also used as a preventative for migraine headaches. While the alkaloid itself doesn't get you high, one can safely assume it has a role in the entourage effect in Opium.

Thebaine

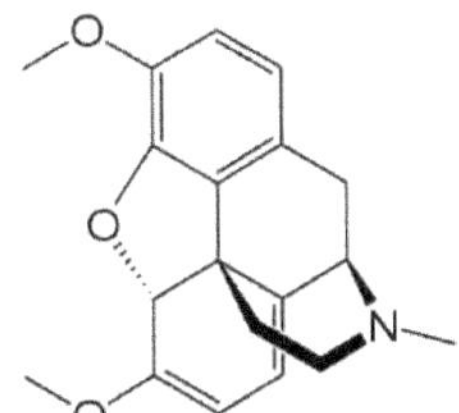

Thebaine is named after Egypt's famously powerful, and possibly first, brand of Opium, *Opium Thebaicum*. Discovered by Thiboumery in 1835, she is chemically similar to both morphine and codeine, yet is stimulatory rather than depressant. This may account for the motivation one feels while under Opium's influences. Thebaine is the alkaloid they convert to make synthetic opioids like Oxycodone. To clear her name, she is also the opiate they use to make Naxalone, the medication that can stop an overdose in its tracks. Yes, the medicine that can prevent an opiate overdose is derived from Opium herself.

Why Opium feels stronger than our natural endorphins

A new study done by scientists out of U.C. San Francisco shows that the opiates in Opium do more than bind to opioid receptors on the surface of cells, as our endogenous opioids do.[7] Their research shows that the reason Opium pleasure is more intense than any natural pleasure is that her opiates bind also to opioid receptors *inside* the cells, which our endorphins cannot do. When researchers applied Morphine to a nerve cell it quickly crossed the cell membrane. Within 20 seconds the Morphine had bound to receptors in an internal cell structure known as the Golgi apparatus, lighting up the internal as well as the external opioid receptors. It has been long believed that when opioid receptors are taken inside the cell to compartments called endosomes, they no longer signal. Instead, these scientists learned that when Morphine crossed the cell membrane the receptors became active from within the cell, receptors that our endogenous opioids can't even get to let alone set off. Opium's alkaloids can and do, causing at least twice the bang for the buck.

Science - A Deadly Necessity

Synthetic and Semi-Synthetic Opiates

Man has an unbridled obsession with the mechanics of things. We feel the need to deconstruct everything to see what makes it tick. We break it down and lay its parts out on the table. We find what makes it work and, once that's done, we just know that we can make it better. It's not even a question of *if*. The only question that comes to mind is *how much better, stronger, and faster can we make it?* It's part of what makes us human. That need to improve upon everything has led to many great things.

We have the ultimate shelters to separate us from wildlife, allowing us privacy to do, well, the same shit the wildlife is doing, but in private. We can travel at speeds that no other living creature can, making this planet we live on, and even our solar system, relatively small. Instead of hunting or grazing, we can have food delivered to our door. No need to seek out water when we have it on tap and in bottles. We watch other humans pretend to live the lives that we wish we had access to, and we do this on giant screens in what we ironically call a *living* room. And why not have a living room, considering we are living longer than ever before? But we can even improve on that. A new supplement has slowed the aging process in mice, extending their life span by 24%.[8] Guess who's taking that pill next.

But all this progress comes at the cost of the world we live in. While we improve our lives in the short term, we rape the planet we live on, making it uninhabitable for not only the wildlife that we so blatantly disregard but, ultimately, for ourselves. The natural world is shrinking while our homes are getting bigger. Our cities grow as we destroy what little remains of nature. As we enjoy the pleasures of modern technology at our fingertips, the earth heats up to a fever, trying to shake us like a virus.

What we call a life makes absolutely no sense in the natural world. Since the Industrial Revolution, we have transformed the Earth into an unrecognizable version of itself. For the first time in our history, we can see our cities from space and yet, even in the darkest locations on the planet, we can no longer look into the sky to see the galaxy we live in. It is perfectly legal to kill anything we deem a bother to our daily lives while it is illegal to grow certain plants, and only because someone decided that it is somehow wrong to eat something that alters our perception of their reality. Happiness must come from within unless big pharma gets a taste of the profits. Progress comes at a price. That statement is even true of our conquest of pain.

In his book, *Opium for the Masses*, author and Opium enthusiast Jim Hogshire writes that "Opium is the mother of all analgesics. There is not much pain that can withstand the effects of opium." Truer words have never been spoken. Since Friedrich Serturner first isolated Morphine from the Opium poppy, scientists have been working to *improve* upon its natural design. All Opiates, natural, semi-synthetic, and synthetic, are derived from alkaloids that are produced by the Papaver Somniferum plant. By isolating the very first *active ingredient*, ol' Freddy had set in motion the end of herbal medicines. Doctors would soon have more powerful remedies to prescribe, forcing us to all but forget the powers of nature's symbiotic relationship with its inhabitants. With the help of Opium, Opium as a natural remedy has been made obsolete.

70 years after Opium's first alkaloid was isolated, English chemist and founder of the Royal Institute of Chemistry C. R. Alder Wright

synthesized the first opiate that does not occur naturally, diacetylmorphine. The drug didn't gain popularity until it was re-synthesized 23 years later by chemist Felix Hoffmann, who also synthesized a chemically pure and stable form of Aspirin for the Bayer pharmaceutical company. In an attempt to make Codeine from Morphine, Felix had instead made diacetylmorphine. The resulting product was twice as strong as its natural counterpart, Morphine. The folks at Bayer were so happy that they named their new drug after the German word for heroic and strong. They called it Heroin.

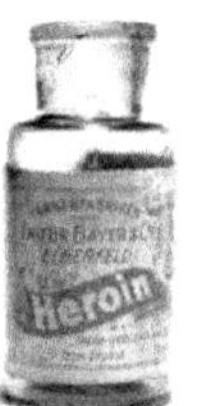

Before it was a word associated with street drugs and junkies, before it was the scourge of society, Heroin was an over-the-counter drug that was marketed by Bayer as a non-addictive alternative to Morphine, which was a popular recreational drug at the time. They couldn't have been more wrong. Heroin is not only twice as strong as Morphine but also that much more addictive as well. By playing with nature to find a cheaper and easier way to isolate an Opium alkaloid, Bayer catapulted the opioid epidemic to new heights.

Chemists kept trying to make an opiate that was less dangerous and addictive than their naturally occurring cousins, each time failing and each time creating a monster that was progressively stronger and more deadly. Oxymorphone in 1914 followed by oxycodone in 1916, both semi-synthetics created by German chemists trying to find something less addictive than Morphine, and each more addictive than the last.

The first fully synthetic opioid was meperidine, later known as Demerol, by German chemist Otto Eisleb in 1932. Then came methadone in 1937. In 1959 Fentanyl, which is 100 times more powerful and deadly than Morphine, was developed by Belgian physician Paul Jansen. Etonitazene, first reported in 1957, followed by Etorphine, synthesized in 1960, are both 1,000 to 3,000 times the strength of Morphine. The latter is used to immobilize elephants while the former is arguably the most addictive substance on Earth.

To give you a reference to how addictive Etonitazene actually is, I'll tell you the story of Thomas K. Highsmith. A chemist at the prestigious laboratory Morton Thiokol, in 2003 he started secretly manufacturing etonitazene for personal use. It wasn't long before he was at its mercy or lack thereof. He would show up for work snorting a 12-ounce spray bottle of his product throughout the day. In a matter of months, he was taking 300 times his original dose. When a coworker became suspicious of Highsmith's behavior, they reported him to the law. By that time, his addiction was about that of 500 bags of heroin a day. Before his court date, he took his own life to escape the pain of withdrawal.

Then there is the case of pharaoh fentanyl, which a Canadian man began experimenting with in order to make some extra cash. His curiosity got the better of him and, before long, he was taking almost 700 times his original dose. His habit was the equivalent of 3,300 bags of heroin a day, which he quit cold turkey. According to Hamilton Morris, a leading researcher in the study of psychoactive substances, "His breath alone was strong enough to make someone nod."[9]

And if you think that this is getting fucking ridiculous, you're right. It's hard to even fathom that a drug known only as 4-F-Ohmefentanyl is about 18,000 times as strong as Morphine. And you thought Heroin was bad. This shit makes Demerol look like aspirin. It's hard for me to wrap my head around the high, the thought making me sick to my stomach. I can only imagine how good that would feel, if only for a moment, and likely my last. Cleopatra would have been jealous.

Today, there are almost 150 synthetic opioids. In the search to create a drug that is less deadly and less addictive, science has made drugs that can relieve even the worst pain imaginable. The focus has become less about making a safe alternative to Opium and more about increasing its strength and power. Both the means and the ends seem futile. After all their attempts, none are less addictive and less deadly than Opium. In fact, the more potent an Opiate is, the more addictive and deadly it is.

On the positive side, the isolation of alkaloids led to many beneficial discoveries. Opium's potency varies, yet by isolating Morphine it became possible to regulate dosage. To that end, doctors are able to administer the amount needed without it being too weak to work or too potent to survive. In addition, the study of opioids and their receptors in the brain brought scientists down a road that led to medications such as anti-depressants, anti-psychotics, and other personality and mood-stabilizing discoveries.

The Entourage Effect Part II

Opium is not simply a source of alkaloids to be extracted, purified, synthesized, or otherwise manipulated by man to achieve his goal of perfecting on Nature. It is a naturally occurring alkaloid cocktail that can be used to relieve anything from pain, cough, and diarrhea to erectile dysfunction, depression, and anxiety. It works as both a stimulant and a depressant, causing periods of relaxation with simultaneous stimulation, making it a wonderful motivational and recreational substance. In other words, this wonder cure can treat whatever ails you while making you both chill and productive, the only downside being lifelong dependence if you're not careful and don't respect its rules.

Each of the alkaloids in Opium has a separate, yet sometimes overlapping, effect on the body and mind. In various combinations, they do different things, just like our own brain chemistry. Even the alkaloids that seem to have no medical value on their own are likely working in conjunction with their constituents. And then there are some opiates that counteract the adverse effects of others. Singly, opiates cause symptoms and side effects that Opium does not.

One might argue that these alkaloids were never meant to be separated from their original formula. They are together by design and best used in nature's recipe. In its purest form, Opium is the perfect medicine. Man's quest to outsmart the natural world is thwarted by his belief that he can do so. Man's need to control nature in the name of *progress* is both beneficial to mankind and detrimental to him and to the ways of the natural world. By that token, Opium is both the cure and the disease, while man is both the innovator and the destroyer of all things.

What's all the yelling about?

With the birds we share this lonely view - RHCP

What Opium feels like

In his memoir, *Confessions of an English Opium Eater*, Thomas De Quincey described the feeling of Opium as follows.

...in an hour, O heavens! what a revulsion! what a resurrection, from its lowest depths, of the inner spirit! what an apocalypse of the world within me! that my pains had vanished was now a trifle in my eyes; this negative effect was swallowed up in the immensity of those positive effects which had opened before me, in the abyss of divine enjoyment thus suddenly revealed. Here was a panacea ... for all human woes; here was the secret of happiness, about which philosophers had disputed for so many ages, at once discovered; happiness might now be bought for a penny and carried in the waistcoat pocket; portable ecstasies might be had corked up in a pint-bottle; and peace of mind would be sent down by mail.

Unless you have personally experienced an Opium high, it's not likely that anyone could author a description that would truly describe how it feels. It would be like explaining orgasms to the chaste. No other feeling on earth is similar in comparison. While it might be tempting to say that it feels like a few glasses of wine while smoking a joint of the finest weed, Opium can't be weighed against other intoxicants with any real value. Even if one were to find the perfect combination of substances, to use those references they would be relying on the reader to have prior experience with that precise recipe. No, there is no way to describe the feeling of Opium. That said, I think I'll give it a try.

The Opium high feels like being pet by God. A warmth spreads over the face and washes down the rest of the body like a shower of bliss. Worry and anxiety fall away so gently that you don't remember them ever being a part of your consciousness in the first place. Life's aches, both physical and otherwise, relent, giving way to a sense of immortality not experienced since youth. Bliss accompanies euphoria, creating a mood that is comparable to the first time you fell in love. Complete mental and physical relaxation contrasts perpetual motivation, complimented by an enhanced sense of well-being. In other words, you feel fucking awesome.

Focus is another happy side effect of Opium and other opiates. Unlike Cannabis, which takes you away from your original point, dragging you down different rabbit holes of thought until you've forgotten where it was that you began, Opium can focus the mind on a singular idea and help you find your way through the maze. One thing that I have noticed with heroin addicts is their uncanny ability to nod out in mid-sentence. The strange part is that when they *wake up* several minutes later, they finish their thoughts as if no time has elapsed. The mind is truly focused, even when it can't be.

At higher doses, as with all of Opium's derivatives, one nods off or enters a dream state between consciousness and sleep. This is where Opium dreams take place and *hallucinations* begin. Hallucination, however, is a strong word that I feel doesn't apply here. In my experience, hallucinations happen in a fully wakened state such as that of a PCP trip. Even LSD hallucinations are more of an altered perception. In an Acid trip, or one of more natural means such as mushrooms, ordinary visual stimulations change and move in a way that wouldn't ordinarily do so. On a PCP trip, one has true hallucinations and sees things that aren't based in reality. It's as if you are in a waking dream. Reality falls away and the dream becomes what is real. With Opium, you simply fall in and out of a dream, like when you nod out at work. This is not a true hallucination. It is a dream, or a daydream at best.

And while an Opium dream is not what I consider a true hallucination, it's as real as any dream you have ever had. What makes it better than a sleeping dream is that you can usually remember what was happening upon waking. This is the fuel that inspired the writings of authors like Percy and Mary Shelley, Edgar Allen Poe, and Charles Dickens, and the character creations of such greats as Bella Lugosi's Dracula. Don't think you'll see little green men after a batch of Opium tea. If you're lucky, you may experience a movie of the mind.

Still, we need to be careful. Aside from problems with addiction, which I will get into later, there is a serious risk of overdose. Opium is 10% to 20% Morphine, as well as about 5% Codeine. There are also other alkaloids, in various percentages, that can add to potential problems. Between 60 and 200 milligrams of Morphine, on its own, can cause a fatal overdose. Just two grams of pure Opium can contain those 200 milligrams in addition to 100 milligrams of Codeine. Someone who has no built-up tolerance to opiates can accidentally take a fatal dose of Opium. As with any medicinal plant you have never tried, less is more.

CHAPTER 3

THE WORLD'S FIRST MEDICINE – A HISTORY OF OPIUM

History

Personal History (Part 1)

My personal history with opiates goes back to the mid-1980s. I was 13 when my best friend, who I refer to as the Phantom due to his ability to appear and disappear in social situations without notice, told me his older brother was a drug dealer and that I needed to try "speed." It was 8th grade, and it was lunchtime. I figured *what the fuck* and I took my first pill. As I later discovered, my pal wasn't the brother of a dealer, he was just an excellent bullshit artist. Not only did he not have an older brother, which I wouldn't learn for many years to come, but he had no idea what pill he was feeding us at any given moment.

The fact was, Phantom had a bag with many different tablets of all shapes and sizes that he gave our group. He was using us, in the way that labs use rats, to figure out the effects of each of them. One pill made us urinate relentlessly while another seemed to have no effect, other than to make our faces flush and warm. One pill makes you larger and the other makes you small, and the ones he stole from his mother did everything and all. After some trial and error, we eventually found our glass slipper and it fit perfectly.

One of the girls in our little crew brought to school a pharmaceutical book known as *The Physician's Desk Reference*, complete with pictures, from her doctor dad's collection. It was a must-have for anyone raiding medicine cabinets before internet search engines. These days you can simply type the color, shape, and markings into any search engine and see what the medication is, what it does, the dosage and side effects, and so on. Pre-internet, unless you had a book such as this, taking pills that weren't prescribed to you was mostly guesswork. Trial and error could kill you and trusting the knowledge of whomever handed you the pill you were about to take was even more dangerous when you had a friend like the Phantom.

We decided to look for the one pill that made us mellow and down, yet alert and talkative. It was total euphoria, the only side effect being a constant itch that made us scratch until we bled. This pill made us feel like we imagined life should feel like every day. Pure bliss, other than hacking away at our flesh to relieve the itch. As she turned one of the pages an image jumped out at me, and there it was, Empirim 4. We were eating codeine, not speed. While his lie was never more apparent, we weren't the slightest bit mad. From that pill, we felt happier and more confident than we ever had before.

Prior to this, my experience with sensory-altering substances was limited to alcohol and weed. In the coming years, I would experiment with and master many more of these gifts of nature, favoring mostly psychedelics. Still, many incarnations of opiates and their derivatives made their way across my path, constantly tempting me to make them an everyday part of my life. This I resisted for two main reasons. First, I could see how I could fall in love with such a thing and be caught in its grips. I didn't care to want or need anything all the time, and that desire to remain free was amplified by my second reason.

Many years later, while sitting in a cell of my own invention pondering the miscalculations that led me astray, I was contemplating the possibilities of my recent past when a frail man entered and staggered to his bunk. He was but a skin-covered skeleton, so thin that one could count the bones that made up his meager frame. Ace bandages around his ankles and wrists gave the only support that the muscles that had faded away were supposed to. It was here that the heroin addict told me the drug dealer's motto. *The first day,* he whispered, *I'm your friend. The second day, I'm your best friend. The third day, I'm your dealer.*

While I avoided them when I could, I always knew that opiates were my true love. And for good reason, which I will get into further on. I, instead, turned my attention to psychedelics and the less ostracized and equally destructive alternative, alcohol. The latter gave the same feeling of confidence and elation. The psychedelics, on the other hand, gifted *us* with spiritual experiences without the guilt and Dogma of an organized religion. With those, *we* transversed space and time, breaking through the *reality* and hypocrisy of society, thus forming *our* own *world* in which *we* lived for a time. But that, my friends, is another story altogether. One I will tell at a later date, for this story is about Opium.

A Brief History - Opium in Antiquity and Beyond

Papaver Somniferum was first classified by Carl Linnaeus in his *Species Plantarum,* or The Species of Plants, in 1753. However, the true history of all Opium began thousands of years before old Carl ever put pen to paper. Our ancestors used opium for pain relief and pleasure long before they learned to scratch crude symbols into stone and clay. In fact, Opium was being used before words were ever spoken. Neanderthals inhabited the Mediterranean, where the Opium poppy is thought to have originated, at least 300,000 years ago. Fossil evidence shows Stone Age hunter-gatherers found their way to Europe a million years ago and evidence of modern human presence in the Mediterranean dates to at least 9,000 years ago. And if you don't think these *cavemen* were partaking in the dope, you'd be sadly mistaken.

Our ancestral use of opiates can be surmised from the fact that wild animals raid opium fields on a regular basis. While crop circles are usually blamed on visitors from another planet, or vandals trying to fool the public, in Australia they are caused by doped-up wildlife. Wallabies in Tasmania, the supplier of half of the world's *legally* grown opium, are known to raid poppy fields to catch a buzz. Once they start to feel it, they hop and graze in circles before passing out. Once they have discovered the alkaloid-rich food source, they regularly come back for more.

Sheep that are allowed to graze in the same fields after a harvest is cleared, eat whatever leftovers they can find. They then play follow the leader in large circles, just like the wallabies. Why it makes these animals graze in looping patterns is unknown, but I'd guess that it's because they're high as fuck. Each animal seems to love Poppies as much as the next. Wild deer have been reported to act strangely in the poppy fields of Tasmania, according to the operations manager of a company called Tasmanian Alkaloids. The deer seem to act strangely and are not as afraid of humans as they normally are. Cockatoos in the area also raid the fields daily, right around harvest time.

In case you're thinking it's a local phenomenon, this behavior isn't exclusive to Tasmania. Flocks of wild parrots in central India, specifically in the Madhya Pradesh state, have been captured on video ripping apart Papaver Somniferum pods. In some cases, they are seen cutting the stems below the seed pods and flying away with the best part, taking the pods back to their nests for consumption. They have even learned to avoid detection by silently swooping down to collect their favorite alkaloid-rich plants. Even ducklings have been shown to ignore their mother's calls while eating opium poppies. Human teenagers exhibit similar behavior when exposed to psychoactive plants, but that's another issue altogether. It should also be noted that the overdose rate of wildlife raiding poppy fields and eating as much as they want is zero percent.

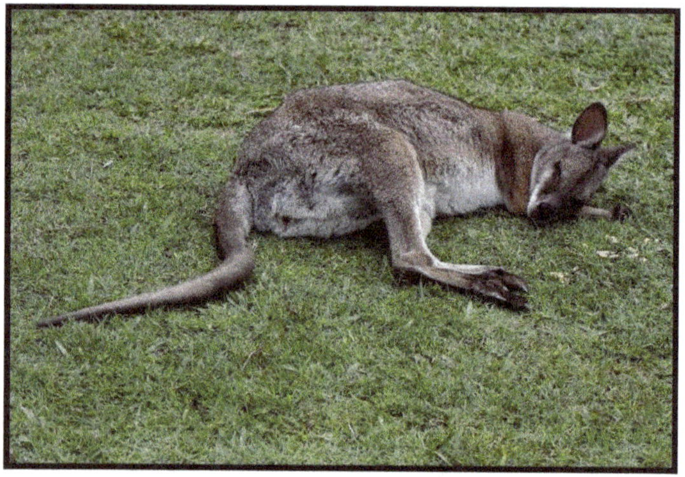

Wallaby catching a nod

It's barely a stretch of the imagination to think that our ancestors, without the hypocritical rules of modern society and yet all the curiosity of a stranger in a strange land, began regular use of Opium from the moment they happened upon the beautifully flowering plant all those millennia ago. If wild animals can figure out which plant gives them euphoric energy, and they go back again and again, what would make anyone think that our ancestors didn't do the same? The question isn't whether early hominoids used Opium for pleasure, and to relieve pain and other ailments. The question is *why is there a plant that mimics our body's own pain management and reward center?* For what natural reason would a plant contain alkaloids that work so specifically on the central nervous systems of most animals?

While the jury is still out, there are three main theories about why the Opium poppy evolved its *magic* ingredients in the first place. One proposes that it evolved naturally, as a deterrent to protect the species from wildlife. This theory appears to be an oversimplification, at the very least. The alkaloids in Papaver Somniferum don't seem to deter deer, sheep, wallabies, ducklings, or any other animal for that matter. Another theory surmises that this beautiful flowering plant was bred by those same *cave-dwelling* ancestors of ours from other ancient poppies that contained lower concentrations of opiate alkaloids for the express purpose of obtaining the strongest alkaloid content possible.

A third theory, and possibly my favorite, is that Papaver Somniferum evolved Opium for the distinct purpose of ensuring a symbiotic relationship with our ancestors. This theory suggests that the alkaloids in Papaver Somniferum exist solely so that evolved primates would cultivate the plant, ensuring its survival. In other words, she gets us high so we will take care of her. Based on the fact that the world now produces about 2000 tons of Opium a year, I'd say that relationship is working well for both parties. The final theory, which was completely undisputed until Hippocrates came along about 2400 years ago, is that Opium is a magical gift from the God(s). Whichever theory you align yourself with, Opium *is* a gift of nature that happens to work like no other plant on the planet. It is the *only* source of Morphine, other than what organisms like us make internally.

Of over 250 species of Papaver, only Papaver Somniferum and Papaver Bracteatum produce alkaloids in any significant amount, the latter containing no Morphine. Papaver Bracteatum does, however, contain high concentrations of Thebaine which is used to make semisynthetic Opiates like Oxycodone, Hydrocodone, Oxymorphone, and more. Thebaine is also used to make Naloxone, which is successfully used to reverse opiate overdoses. Of all the species of Papaver, of any plant in the entire plant kingdom, only Papaver Somniferum produces Morphine.

The earliest evidence for human use and cultivation of opiates dates back some 8000 years or so to a site in La Marmotta in Italy during the Neolithic period. Radiocarbon dating of 22 samples from sites around Europe shows the Opium poppy was present in the Mediterranean since at least 5622 BCE where it may have grown naturally (no one really knows Somniferum's origin for sure) and was cultivated by Neolithic communities. It was almost immediately dispersed outside of its native area, first to the west of the Rhine in around 5300 BCE and then to the western Alps by about 5000 BCE. In other words, man was cultivating Papaver Somniferum, taking it with him from place to place and planting it hundreds of miles away, at the very least since the dawn of Western civilization.

Traces of a Poppy capsule were also found in the teeth of a skeleton buried over 6000 years ago in Barcelona, Spain. Evidence even suggests that Neanderthals used Opium some 30,000 years ago. Archeological sites prove that the seeds spread to Europe and other areas surrounding the Mediterranean where they were not native. This was not by some accident of nature. This was agriculture. Opium poppies have been found at a minimum of 17 sites in Neolithic settlements throughout Switzerland, Germany, and Spain, including a large number of seeds in a container at a 4,200-year-old burial site in Spain. This can only mean that, during the Stone Age, Neolithic people were cultivating and sharing opium poppies.

The earliest written account of Opium use comes from Mesopotamia around 4500 years ago. Not so coincidentally, the first *prescription* for Opium was found in the exact place (*and around the same time*) that written language is believed to have been invented. The ancient Sumerians, the potential inventors of literacy itself, wrote of the plant that they called *Hul Gil*, or "*the joy plant*." They obviously used the poppy recreationally, falling in love with its mind and body-altering properties, and immediately felt the need to leave a record of this powerful medicine for future generations, just as soon as they figured out a way to write.

In the eighth to seventh century B.C.E., Homer wrote of Opium in the Odyssey writing "...she sipped a drug that had the power of robbing grief and anger of their sting and banishing painful memories." Around the same time, Poppy Juice was also described in the seventh century B.C.E. on Assyrian medical tablets in the royal library of Babylonian King Assurbanipal. These tablets are thought to be copies of earlier texts. The Kahun Papyrus of Egypt, one of the oldest surviving medical texts dated to 1800 B.C.E., prescribes Opium for pain. In the Ebers Papyrus, from about 1550 B.C.E., and also in the four oldest surviving medical texts, Opium is included in hundreds of remedies including one to sedate children. The same remedy the goddess Isis was fabled to use to sedate her son, Horus.

Demeter, or *Mother Earth*, is the Greek goddess of agriculture and the harvest. Written about from at least 1400 to 1200 B.C.E., she is also known as the Poppy Goddess, and for good reason. The sister and consort of Zeus, together they had a daughter named Persephone whom Zeus allowed her uncle Hades to abduct and marry. When Demeter heard the news, she began to search the world for her daughter, not knowing she was already in the underworld. In her search, she came upon a place called Mekone. It was there that she learned that drinking the sap of the Poppy immediately relieved her of her anguish.

Demeter forced Zeus to make Hades agree to return Persephone, but before he did, he fed her Pomegranates. Having eaten of the underworld (pomegranates are from Hades, apparently), Persephone had to return to Hades for one-third of every year. For that time, Demeter would drink the juice of the Poppy and sleep. The months leading up to her daughter leaving caused Demeter to become sad and withdrawn, thus causing Autumn as the goddess of harvest began to grieve. With the help of the Opium Poppy, she slept, bringing the death of winter. Upon her daughter's return, Demeter would awaken, and spring would begin. In commemoration of this, Demeter is depicted in statues with Poppies in hand and on her headdress. She even metamorphosed her human lover, Mecon (or Mekon), into a Poppy plant.

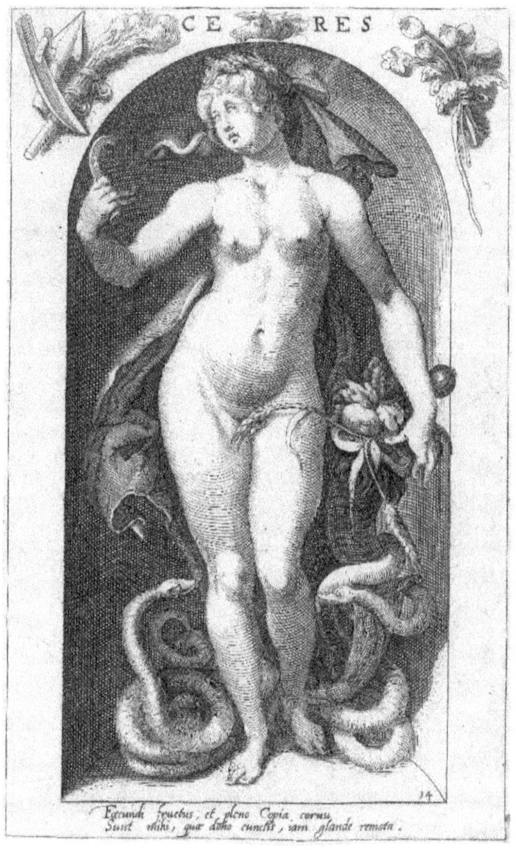

Demeter (Haarlem, 1598)
Karel van Mander

Hippocrates, the father of medicine and the originator of the Hippocratic Oath that all physicians must swear by, believed that

Opium was man's best medicine. He believed that disease, being naturally caused, should be treated with nature's medicine. Being a logical man, he disassociated himself with the magical attributes given to Opium. He, instead, saw it as the natural medicine that it is and prescribed it for several ailments. He also knew of the dangers of Opium abuse and cautioned that it should be used sparingly. Even Theophrastus, the successor of Aristotle, author of Historia Plantarum (History of Plants) and the other father of botany, also wrote of Opium (or Opion) in 300 B.C.E.

The Romans saw the many benefits of Opium, as well as some dark uses. To them, it was a religious enhancement, a painkiller, and a convenient poison. It could quietly take the life of an enemy, as well as peacefully end one's own. Hannibal, not the cannibal of the Thomas Harris novel but the Carthaginian general and one of the greatest military commanders in history, kept a lethal dose in a small chamber in his ring, which he is said to have used to end his own life between 183 and 181 B.C.E.

It wasn't until the 1300s A.D. that the king of Thailand prohibited the use of Opium, something no government had ever thought necessary prior. That only lasted for 500 years. The British overturned anti-opium laws when they colonized parts of Burma, seeing an opportunity to capitalize on the plant by regulating its sale. They then enacted the Pharmacy Act of 1868, limiting the sale of poisons and narcotics to qualified pharmacists and druggists. Still, Opium and its products were sold over the counter. It wasn't until the Dangerous Drug Act of 1920 that opiates, and coca products required a prescription.

For 6,000 years of historically recorded use (and 30,000 years of archeologically proven use), opium was legally given, traded, or sold to whoever desired its properties. Its access has only been controlled in the U.K. for around 100 years. In the United States, Opium was technically legal until 50 years ago until the passing of the 1970 Controlled Substance Act. Therefore Opium, which is proven to have been used for pleasure and pain relief for at least

8,000 years and quite possibly since the dawn of time, has only been a controlled substance for little more than 50 of those years.

In 1871-72 Poppy cultivation had grown to over 560,000 acres, and over 10.3 million dollars a year. The equivalent in today's dollar would be 238 million, but that's nothing compared to the 7 billion dollar-a-year opiate market of today. It's even more interesting when you factor in that Opium was legal in 1870 and could be obtained without the need for a prescription. But, like everything that makes a considerable profit in this world, then came the government regulations. Since the regulations began the dollar amount sold per year is 3,000% of what it was in 1871. Factoring for world population increase that is still 500% more opiate dollars per person on the planet. Regulations have been ineffective in slowing opiate use. All they do is guarantee that the governments of the world get their slice of the pie.

In 1880, not long after the popularization of Morphine as an isolated alkaloid, The U.S. and Qing Dynasty China made an agreement prohibiting the shipment of Opium between the countries. Within ten years, the rate of opiate addiction rose from less than one addict per 1000 to almost 5 per 1000 (there's that magic 500% again). Telling people that they can't have something makes them want it more, and this was proven by one of the first prohibitory laws. These laws, made in the guise of helping save people from themselves, were only to control who could make opiates in a successful attempt to make them more profitable. This can be seen in the opioid epidemic of late, and the addiction and death caused by such powerful laboratory-made pharmaceutical-grade opioid derivatives, such as Fentanyl which is 100 times more powerful than Heroin.

Left in a natural setting, opiate deaths would be virtually nonexistent. The work it takes to grow poppies for personal use, harvest them, and naturally extract the intoxicating opiates is not a quick and easy task. The resulting product is far less deadly and addictive and, when used alongside a plan of rules that should never be broken, can be beneficial to the quality of existence, both mentally and physically. Pain can be regulated, and mood elevated. One can be motivated or helped to rest.

The Big O - Opium as an Aphrodisiac

Opium, as we can see from our story of Percy and Mary Shelley, is an excellent aphrodisiac. As charming as Percy was, it wasn't his magnetism alone that made him such an accomplished cocksman. The guy lived a hedonistic lifestyle while maintaining a small harem and still managed to have a few women on the side, each of them professing their love for him until his end or theirs, and beyond. His views on free love were shared by his lovers, even through bouts of jealousy, and made his promiscuity almost acceptable. It wasn't one-sided either. He endured and sometimes encouraged Mary's affairs as well, even if she didn't always act on them. Still, he seemed to be taking advantage of the arrangement more than the others.

How can one man bring that many women to fall so madly in love with him that they don't mind sharing? An adventurous lifestyle helps, but that's not enough. Youth is definitely a factor, as a lot of young men and women are rather experimental at that age (think high school and college). To be young, wild, and carefree could sustain the magic for a time, but not for long. Percy had some help in his endeavors. Don't get me wrong. I'm sure he was one seductive motherfucker, but that's only part of the equation. Endogenous opioid peptides such as endorphins (remember the Morphine within?) play a strong role in forming stable relationships, such as pair bonding (or, in this case, triad bonding) and attachment. Morphine, along with other alkaloids in Opium, does the same.

Opium acts on the central nervous system with several benefits. In moderate doses, it makes one more open to erotic suggestion. It stimulates the libido in both sexes, encouraging blood flow to both the penis and clitoris. This could be the result of Papaverine, which is used to treat erectile dysfunction. Opium also acts with anesthetic properties on the nerves of the penis, vagina, and anus.

This has several desirous effects. With no loss of pleasure, it makes a man last longer which, if you're interested in your partner's experience, can make for a fun night that often ends long after you see the sun peeking through the blinds. Alcohol can have a similar effect, yet it causes drowsiness and has the unpredictable consequence of erectile dysfunction, also known as whiskey dick.

Opium delays the female orgasm as well, without taking away from the pleasure of sexual intercourse. The added bonus of anesthetizing the rectal tissue, according to author Mary Jane Superweed[10], can be "used to make anal intercourse easier." While moderate doses enhance sexual desire, too much can lower the libido, potentially causing you and your date to nod out to some music and just dream about having sex. While this can still be fun, the intention of an aphrodisiac is usually to seal the deal. So here we have an alkaloid cocktail that not only makes you horny as hell but can also mimic the chemicals in our own brains that cause us to fall in love.

This doesn't mean Opium is going to make someone fall in love with you if they aren't already on that path. In fact, it definitely will not. Desire starts with mutual admiration, both of one's physical appearance and of one's spirit. One can be no more convinced to love someone that they do not as they can be persuaded to crave a food that makes them want to gag. There is no magic love potion, number 9 or otherwise. But if the circumstances are right, and a hot spark already exists, Opium can help that fire burn high well into the night and beyond.

No means no. NEVER give anyone anything that they don't know they are taking, and always make sure they are just as into it as you. Drugging someone to gain their sexual desire is not only morally wrong, but it's illegal and, quite frankly, gross and looserish. Sex with someone who doesn't want to have sex with you is far less exciting than masturbation. If someone doesn't want you, do the right thing and go rub one out in the privacy of your room and move on. Putting your energy into someone who doesn't share your vision is energy wasted that could be used to find someone who does. There is no sex that is better than that of mutual desire. Opium can enhance that feeling, but it cannot create it.

CHAPTER 4
SIDE EFFECTS

Nausea and stomach tightening

The first side effect of Opium and all her derivatives is nausea. Your stomach tightens and you feel like you want to puke. The easiest way to make sure this doesn't happen is to eat a full meal before you take it. This is in direct contradiction to the earlier mentioned way of making the experience stronger. In my opinion, it's better to eat and not deal with the need to throw up than it is to puke up your Opium. That said, it can be a rewarding experience to throw up from dope. It can also be your body's way of telling you that you've taken more than you can handle. Another trick is to eat shortly after you take Opium before the nausea sets in.

On a side note, the first time I experienced Heroin I projectile vomited while scratching my arms raw. It wasn't an unpleasant experience, but that was likely due to the fact that I was higher than I had ever been in my long history of drug use. I do not recommend Heroin as a recreational drug. It's way too addictive and deadly and feels so very awesome that I didn't try it again for several years out of fear that I would forever be entangled in its web of destruction. I knew from the first taste, even while puking and scratching, that I was already in love. More could only make it worse. Opium is more subtle and more easily controlled.

Paralyzed bowel

Perhaps the most annoying side effect of Opium, other than addiction, is a paralyzed bowel. It sounds a lot scarier than it actually is. Opium slows the digestive system and causes paralytic ileus. This can be remedied in the same ways constipation is usually remedied, high intake of fiber and, in worse cases, a laxative or stool softener. Metamucil crackers work wonders for intermediate users. Just eat two before you take Opium and two the next morning. Coffee's stimulant properties, in conjunction with a high fiber intake, are all but guaranteed to get you off the bowl sooner.

Difficulty Urinating

Another sometimes annoying side effect of opiates is difficulty urinating. I've read that you can solve this by tickling your ass, but I think there is a better way. There are two urethral sphincters, the external and the internal. The external urethral sphincter is the one you normally use to stop yourself from peeing your pants on a long car ride. The internal urethral sphincter is controlled by the autonomic nervous system, which is thought to be beyond conscious control. The latter is the one that causes *stage fright* when trying to pee in public.

One of the problems with not being able to release the flow of urine is that you are thinking about it. This can lead to anxiety which, in turn, makes it harder to pee. Maybe that's why tickling your ass or rinsing your perineum seems to help. They take your mind off the situation. Some find humming, or other vocalizations, to be helpful as well. I find the best way to regain control is to simply let go of it.

It takes deep concentration to feel which muscle group controls the flow of urine. It's much easier to know what to squeeze when you don't want to piss your pants in public than it is to know which muscles to release when you want the stream to flow. The key is to relax. Specifically, relax the muscles of the pelvic floor. Concentrate on the area just above your mons pubis (where the pubic hair grows) and just below your abs. Let your abs release and let the relaxation flow downward. With some practice, you'll see that it works like magic. Occasionally, you find that when you get distracted the flow will stop suddenly. This only proves that the method is working. Simply relax again. Let it flow and let yourself go.

Delayed Orgasm

The inability to orgasm in a reasonable amount of time as a side effect of Opium use can be a positive, as well as negative. If you want a long night of passionate lovemaking, this is the side effect for you. As mentioned previously, Opium acts as an anesthetic on the reproductive organs, allowing both men and women to delay climax for far more than the average amount of time. If you want to go all night, Opium is your friend. However, if you're looking for a quickie this one will prove to be a hindrance.

WARNING: High probability of chafing.

CHAPTER 5

THE HAND OF DOOM – THE DARK SIDE OF OPIUM

Addiction - The Hand of Doom

So be yearning all your life

Twisting, turning like a knife

- Alice in Chains

Addiction begins naturally from the euphoria that Opium brings. We are genetically designed to love the feeling that Opium produces. As I mentioned earlier, that's because some of the alkaloids made by the Papaver Somniferum plant are the same as substances that are made in our own bodies. These chemicals also mimic the endorphins our own systems make and bind to the very same receptors. So why would nature create a substance in our bodies that not only relieves pain but also makes us happy? Even stranger, why would nature create alkaloids in a plant that does the same thing, only better? Wouldn't it seem more logical that we should have different chemicals that work separate receptors for these two very distinct purposes?

I would argue that it may have played a necessary part in our survival as a species. To help us continue on in the direst of circumstances (imagine a broken leg when you live in the wild) relief from pain may not be enough. One could reason that without the euphoria, and the positive attitude it brings, even a non-life-threatening injury could effectively cause one to give up. Even if a compound fracture to a fibula didn't hurt, it would relieve you of your ability to walk. While that might be all right when you're sitting on your couch watching your flat screen and collecting a disability check, a broken leg in the wild could mean that the hope of survival is all but lost. A bit of a boost in morale could mean the difference between life and death.

Physical Addiction

To stop the sensation of pain from registering, naturally occurring endorphins bind to opiate receptors and block electric pulses from traveling through nerve cells and getting to other parts of the brain. While our naturally occurring endorphins, and even endogenous Morphine, may give us some pain relief and euphoria (while also triggering the release of Dopamine), it's subpar to the effects of Opium. That is partly because, as we learned earlier, Opium's alkaloids can give a hit to receptors that our own chemistry cannot.

The only negative effect of ingesting these externally synthesized medicines is that when we supplement our endorphins with those from an outside source for too long, our bodies self-regulate and slow down the production of endorphins. At the same time, opiates switch off nerve cells called GABAergic neurons, neurons that turn off the euphoria and pleasure networks of the brain, filling the nucleus accumbens with a surge of dopamine and causing happiness and euphoria. When dopamine hits the brain's fear center, the amygdala, stress, and anxiety are washed away.

The GABAergic neurons don't like being blocked from talking to the brain so, over time, they make some adjustments to the body's chemistry in order to get their signals through. They make up to four times as much cyclic adenosine monophosphate (cAMP), a compound that helps these neurons fire electric pulses, in order to compensate for the increase of opiates in the brain. Later, when we stop taking the external opiates, we no longer make enough of the endogenous opiates that we need, and we make way too much of the cAMP. That's when withdrawal begins, and it doesn't stop until our system ramps back up its production.

In the meantime, the body reacts to the sudden lack of exogenous opioids with flu-like symptoms that vary in intensity relative to the strength and frequency of use of the opiate or opiates the user ingested. In other words, the stronger the alkaloid and the more often it is used the stronger the symptoms will be. Someone withdrawing from daily use of, let's say, Fentanyl is much worse than the withdrawal from Opium, and someone who uses a substance several times a day for several months will have much worse symptoms than someone who uses once a day for a few weeks.

The symptoms of withdrawal are almost the exact opposite of the side effects of use. Where opiates cause constipation, withdrawal causes diarrhea. Slowed respiration is now raised blood pressure. Instead of happiness and low stress, we now have depression and anxiety. Mild Opium withdrawal can be as simple as a runny nose and congestion, followed by a bad case of restless leg syndrome at the end of the day, while a severe addiction can be bad enough to cause someone to end their life to escape the pain, as we learned from young Thomas Highsmith and his addiction to Etonitazene. I find it interesting to note that people's last names were at one time given depending on their profession and that the man who was manufacturing one of the most powerful opiates of all time in order to get high was named Highsmith.

Withdrawal symptoms begin between 6 and 48 hours after the last time the substance is ingested. The longer the drug lasts, the longer it can take for the symptoms to begin. The first stage of symptoms can start out mild and increase in intensity as withdrawal progresses. The user begins to feel anxious and irritable. His or her blood pressure begins to increase, and they may run a slight fever. The feeling of a cold coming on is usually dismissed as just that, while congestion, sneezing, and a runny nose begin. The addicted may begin to sweat, and their heart can start to race. Then comes the restless leg and muscle aches that contribute to trouble sleeping. At this point, after hours of staring at the ceiling while shaking that annoying feeling out of one leg or the other, the user often decides to mitigate their symptoms by using just a little bit, *just a taste* of what their body craves.

If the person has the will to make it through the first stage without relapsing, they enter the second phase of withdrawal which can persist from day two until day ten, sometimes longer but rarely. It's likely that the earlier-mentioned symptoms worsen, and new ones arise. Chills run up the spine and out to the ends of the limbs. One can shiver uncontrollably while sharp stomach pain feels like a knife in the belly. To add insult to injury, uncontrollable vomiting is complimented by the inevitable process of shitting oneself. I once had a heroin addict show up at my home wearing only a blanket and asking if he could sleep on my floor in order to hide his mishap from his family. He told me that he drove an hour to New York City's Lower East Side to cop his fix, only to find a high police presence where his dealers usually were. I, of course, obliged and he cleaned up and crashed on my couch. Today he is sober and has been for nearly 20 years. As he can tell you, the cravings at this stage are the most intense one can feel. Anything to end the pain. If you make it through these you are one step closer to the end, but it's not over yet.

The final stage of withdrawal can last for weeks. These symptoms are usually reserved for addicts who have been using them for years in extreme amounts but can be observed in anyone who uses them to the point of never being straight. When you keep yourself high enough for long enough, long-term damage can result. Cravings persist and become all-consuming with an added depression and anxiety that would surely be alleviated by a quick fix. A never-ending fatigue, with insomnia adding to its torture, makes it hard to get out of bed. In some cases, memory loss and extreme emotional outbursts can persist.

Physical withdrawal can be almost completely avoided, if one can exhibit remarkable self-control, by weaning off of whatever opiate you are addicted to. While mild symptoms may be experienced, one can avoid almost all of the pain of the experience by simply lowering their dose daily until they are taking none. Weaning can be done incrementally at whatever dose reduction the user is comfortable with, as long as the dose is reduced every time the opiate is ingested. Lengthening the time between doses can also speed up the process. Weaning is the hardest thing for a true addict to accomplish as it requires access to the substance that they so desire without allowing themselves to do enough to actually feel the high in the way they would like to. While this takes care of the physical addiction, it only teases the chemically addicted brain, leaving one susceptible to relapse at any given point in the process.

Emotional *Addiction*

I'm not, myself, addicted to opiates. That is to say, I have no physical dependence on opium or any of its derivatives. If I don't ingest them, I'm not going to get sick, vomit, or shit myself. I'm not going to steal, or lie, or sell my ass to get a fix. Even if I feel the urge to use, I'm not going to run out and score. I can have painkillers in the medicine cabinet and not take any for days, sometimes weeks, or months. When I need them, I use them as directed (for the most part). The second I no longer have a medical need for them, those same painkillers may become recreational, and all bets are off.

Not being completely physiologically addicted doesn't mean I don't get what's called a *chip*. A chip is a very slight physical dependence that doesn't carry the same weight as full-blown addiction. After a few days of use, symptoms can occur that the user may barely notice if they perceive them at all. One might feel more agitated than they normally do. Simple disagreements can become highly argumentative and curt remarks can seem like complete disrespect. As mentioned earlier, someone with a chip may have trouble sleeping due to restless leg syndrome. One may even be preoccupied with thoughts of Opium and its pleasures. If you are not careful at this stage, giving in to these desires can launch you into a full-blown physical addiction.

I've been completely and hopelessly addicted to a few substances in my life but never opiates. Not at least in the way I was addicted to other *recreationals* over the years. That's because I have great respect for the power of the one thing on the planet intended by nature itself to be our greatest pleasure-inducing medicine. I've seen strong men brought to their knees by Opium's synthetic and semi-synthetic cousins. I've stood over their graves as we mourned their loss. I've learned to control my intake so that, hopefully, she can never control me. I've used Opium to subsidize, and eventually find relief from, an alcohol addiction that I endured for over 20 years. No. I'm not physically addicted to opium or its derivatives. That said, I've been *emotionally* addicted to opiates for over 35 years. But what does it mean to be *emotionally*, or *psychologically* addicted? Well, let me explain.

First of all, I dislike the connotations of the terms *emotional addiction* and *psychological addiction*. While my explanation of addiction will sound both emotional and psychological, it is a chemical addiction in the same way a physical addiction is simply chemically motivated. Therefore, they are the same. Both are caused by substances created in the body and a lack thereof. Both cause one to seek out whatever it is they are addicted to, whether they want to or not. While you may *feel* no physical withdrawal symptoms (such as pain, diarrhea, or vomiting), you definitely feel a need to get that substance into your body as quickly as possible.

For example, I was addicted to cocaine products for about a decade, years after the *fun* of it had subsided. The longer I went without them, the less I felt the need to have them. Still, whenever I was presented with my drug of choice, I didn't have the ability to turn it down. *Just say no* was no longer an option. The stronger the version, the more addictive it was. Powdered cocaine was not a problem for me. I could take it or leave it. Add a little baking soda and water, and some heat from a lighter, and you have freebase (also known as crack). One taste of that and all I could think about was getting more. While I never injected anything recreationally, those whom I saw injecting cocaine were more fiendish and paranoid than crackheads. Something that makes you instantly crave more is not psychological (which is defined as having a mental rather than a physical cause) or emotional, it's chemical.

A species of Carpenter ant lives high in the canopy of tropical forests where it has an extensive network of aerial trails. When it finds gaps in the canopy that are difficult to cross, this ant wanders to the forest floor where it is exposed to a fungus called *Ophiocordyceps unilateralis*. The spores attach to the ant's exoskeleton and eventually break through it. The carpenter ant goes about its business, not knowing it is infected, and returns to its normal behavior of foraging for food and delivering it to the nest, high in the trees above the forest floor. Out of nowhere, the ant begins to experience irregularly timed full-body convulsions that cause it to fall back to the forest floor. Then comes the strange part.

The ant seeks out an area with the right temperature and humidity for the fungus to thrive. When it finds this perfect environment, around 70 to 85 degrees Fahrenheit and 95% humidity, the carpenter ant climbs until it finds a leaf that is almost exactly 10 inches above the ground on the northern side of the plant. It walks the underside of the leaf and with abnormal force uses its mandibles to bite into the leaf vein, at which point it becomes paralyzed in its death grip on the plant. The fungus feeds on the ant until it dies. Mycelia structurally fortify the ant's exoskeleton and grow out of it, attaching it securely to the leaf. Fruiting bodies sprout from the now-dead ant's head to release spores that will eventually find a new host.

While this analogy has a world of differences between itself and addiction, it has similarities that cannot be disputed. Something introduced to these creatures causes them to make choices that they otherwise would not make, choices that are detrimental to their existence, in order to benefit the invader. One could argue that addiction benefits the substance that the user is craving by causing the addict to propagate its source. The addict experiences an illogical need to disregard everything that they love in order to obtain something that may well be destroying their lives. This addiction is no more emotional than what the carpenter ant experiences and I don't think that anyone would say that Zombie ants have a psychological problem.

When you are in love, you can become emotionally addicted to a person. When you are a fan of someone or something, like a band or a celebrity, you can become emotionally addicted to it. When you are obsessed with a particular item, such as a fast car or a lifestyle, you can be emotionally addicted to that thing or idea. You think about it often and crave whatever it is about it that drives you mad. Whatever you long for, you can be emotionally addicted to it. Whatever you may be obsessed with you are addicted to. That's what obsession is. It's an emotional addiction. That's partly because our bodies produce endorphins that activate opiate receptors in the brain. Two of Opium's main constituents, Morphine and Codeine, are endogenous opioids in humans. Nature made us all addicts before we ever knew what addiction was.

To call an addiction psychological or emotional implies that the addict has some flaw that makes them more susceptible than the rest of the population. While this could potentially be true for the reason that some people experiment with substances in their youth and others do not, this is not the case for addiction. I've seen older adults with no history of addiction to alcohol or other recreational psychoactives who have become hopelessly addicted to crack (the smokable version of cocaine also known as freebase) after trying it only once. That is not a psychological or emotional issue, it's a true chemical addiction. The brain itself is transformed in such a way that it works against the conscious will of the user in order to get what it wants.

As I mentioned earlier, opiates switch off GABAergic neurons, filling the nucleus accumbens with a surge of dopamine which then floods into the amygdala, where stress and anxiety are cleansed from the palate of the brain. The brain says *this feeling, right here and now, is how I want to feel forever*. It's what the brain craves. It's why we do the things that make us happy and avoid the things that torture our everyday experience. Only now it's free. We didn't have to work to accomplish this euphoria. The mind takes note of this free reward and begs us for it for the rest of our lives. It's not emotional or psychological. It is a physical transformation of brain chemicals and it's locked in our memory, a part of the brain that has evolved to alter our actions and reactions to situations in order to achieve what opiates give us with little to no effort. Ecstasy.

You're an addict and you don't know it

While, as I have mentioned, I am not physically addicted to opiates, a friend and doctor of psychiatry, whom I'll call Mac, once told me that everything we do in life is for benzodiazepines or opiates. We may not be out in the streets scamming up our next fix but, in a sense, we kind of are. Whatever excites you, whatever you long for when it is not around, whatever you want so badly that you ache for it, is an addiction. Every good thing that has ever happened to you was the result of, and the reason for, your craving for opiates. These wants can become all-consuming, even self-destructive. That's because you are producing virtually the same drugs that dope addicts use, opiates. Your body uses them to reward you in the same way a dog is given a treat, that is when you do something that it deems worthy. Social media, ice cream, sex, all of these cause your body to deliver drugs to you from the reward center of your brain, which has receptors for every high imaginable, including happiness and, as you might imagine by this point, love.

Endorphins

We have all heard the word endorphins. We know that they are strange hormones that make us feel good. We know that these brain chemicals make us happy when we do things like run, play, and have sex. These chemicals in our brains reward us when we are enjoying food, the pleasure of company, and when we accomplish goals in our daily lives. What you may not know is that you are getting a spike of opiates every time you do anything that makes you happy. Everything you enjoy, you enjoy because of your opiate receptors.

The word Endorphin is a portmanteau, meaning it is two words squished together to make a new word with meanings from both. A good example is the word smog, which is a combination of smoke and fog. That no-tell motel you sometimes hide out in is named after a blend of the words motor and hotel. Endorphin comes from endogenous, which means originating within, and Morphine. When you go to the gym and experience that *runner's high* you are getting a fix of that *Morphine from within,* endorphins.

From bugs to birds, from lizards to primates like ourselves, most creatures feel pain. They also have opioid receptors and endorphins. Take for example the Squilla mantis. This species of shrimp, found in the coastal areas of the Mediterranean, violently convulse when shocked. While that may seem obvious, when the same shrimp are injected with Morphine the reaction to the shock is less severe. The more morphine they get, the less they feel the pain. Another example is the American Lobster. If you cut off the walking leg of one of these amazing creatures, his endogenous morphine levels (remember the *Morphine within?*) increase by nearly 50%.

A recent study by evolutionary biologist Gregory Wray of Duke University in Durham, North Carolina suggests that having more of these endorphins is what separated us from our chimpanzee cousins, with whom we share 98% of our DNA. Without getting too technical, we have more of the gene that codes for the protein prodynorphin (see the word Morphine squeezed in there?), a precursor to endorphins. Being that, in addition to mood elevation to pain management, endorphins are responsible for social attachment, bonding, and learning through reinforcement and reward, it makes sense that an increase of 20% would cause us to be more *human*. If that's the case, maybe Opium makes us *more human than human.*

Endorphins and endogenous opiates are designed to work with neural tissue for the purpose of pain relief, euphoria, learning, and bonding. Why, then, would only one plant create substances that not only structurally mimic these mood-elating pain relievers, but also create chemicals that our bodies, and the bodies of many other animals, also synthesize for these purposes? And the similarities between our own endorphins and the chemicals found in Opium don't stop there. Opium, like our own nervous system, creates dozens of unique alkaloids that are similar to what our own body releases when we laugh, connect, eat our favorite foods, fall in love, and have sex.

Life, as we hope it to be, is a constant craving for these naturally occurring chemicals. Every task that brings us a feeling of accomplishment, every deed that brings us closer to a goal, and every joy we have ever had is the result of these endorphins. Evolution has forged this addiction into our biology in order to keep us on the path to survival and prosperity. It's no surprise, then, that we act accordingly. Positive behavior is rewarded with endorphins. Like giving a dog a treat when he behaves, nature gives us a treat when we do the things that she has determined beneficial to our existence. Imagine a dog that could give himself a treat. There would be no more need for obedience. This is the true reason that the powers that be don't want you and me to be able to give ourselves our own rewards.

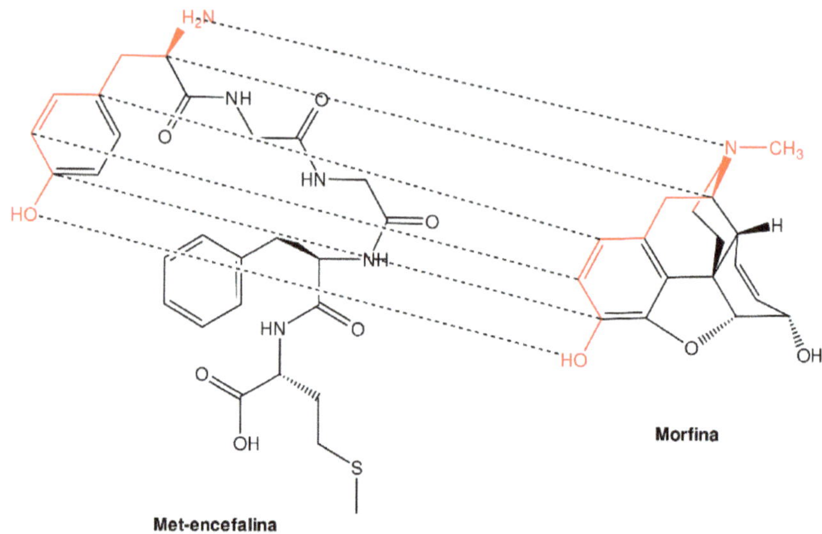

Structural relationship between enkephalins and morphine
"Opioid Peptide." https://en.wikipedia.org/wiki/Opioid_peptide.

The Responsibility of Addiction

Being the addicts that we are born to be comes with a
responsibility. For the same reason you cannot eat cake at every
meal and should probably limit it to birthday parties and other
special occasions, you should be careful of how often you take any
mind-altering substance. That's especially true in the case of
Opium and her derivatives. The love for anything can drive one
mad. The dumbest shit you've done in your life was likely because
you were in love. Retrospectively, you can see how irrational your
actions were and you would never want to repeat the offense. Then
along comes another lover and you find yourself falling into
patterns of behavior that you thought you would never slip into
again. This is what addicts call a relapse.

Everyone has embarrassed themselves in the name of love. None
of us can claim that we never acted the fool when it comes to
attraction. Don't worry. It's not your fault. You were drugged. You

were under the influence of a cocktail of drugs that your body makes, including Oxytocin, Serotonin, and other Endorphins. That's right, Mother Nature slipped you a Mickey. As we learned earlier, endorphins are highly addictive *drugs*. Everything you do, from eating to fucking, is to get a little taste. Without them, sex would feel about as good as rubbing your hands together to keep warm. In the absence of these chemicals even love, the most coveted of all human emotions, could not exist. You're just an addict chasing that high.

Still, addiction has nothing to do with you. That is to say, your conscious thoughts are irrelevant. That's because the part of the body that wants to get high is your brain. Afterward, you may feel regret and guilt. You may swear off alcohol and all psychoactive substances, and you truly intend to keep that promise. That is until the brain sees an opportunity to get a fix. Then, your own mind works against your true wishes, lying to you by convincing you that everything will be fine, even great, if you just get a little high this one time. Your own mind lies to you using your own voice, and how can you not trust yourself, your one and only true ally? And so, you give in. You revel in the excitement of getting the dope, even more in doing it. Then comes the crash, along with the same guilty promises.

In order to stop doing something you have to not want to do it more than you want to do it. I know this sounds confusingly simple but when it comes to drugs and alcohol it's not the same as other problems in life. It's not like you either want to do something or you don't want to do something. You want to do it until it causes a problem and then you don't want to do it ever again. That is, until the problem goes away, at which point you can't wait to do it again. Sometimes the reason you tell yourself that you want to do it again is just to hide from the problem you created by doing it in the first place. The cycle doesn't end until you find control or sink so low that a switch goes off in your brain that sets in motion a desire to escape. Once that desire outweighs the desire to use, the path from addiction begins to reveal itself.

Hand of Doom - The Dark Side of Opium

Oh you, you know you must be blind

To do something like this

To take the sleep that you don't know

You're giving Death a kiss

-Black Sabbath

Opium has all the qualities of a love affair. It makes you feel good. You want it all the time and more and, like any passionate love affair, there's a dark side. When your love betrays you, or they simply stop reciprocating, you want to throw up, and your stomach aches and cramps. You can't sleep due to the fact that as tired as you are, your brain thinks of all the outcomes of every different scenario that could potentially get you back to what you feel you've lost. There are similarities between that feeling and the feeling of a chemical withdrawal. The main difference is that a love lost is much easier to take. I've seen many people discard love when it gets in the way of their addiction.

Unlike other works on the subject that have been published for the masses, I'm not going to candy-coat opiate addiction. I won't downplay it for profit. That would make me no better than your local street dealer. While my passion for Opium has no end, I understand that my love for her is partially, if not completely, the result of some sort of addiction. Long-term use of psychoactive substances causes your natural reward system to get lazy. The pituitary gland works less because your dope is doing its job for him. The fucked-up part is that the dope is doing it better than he is. Even when he comes back to work full-time, you remember how much better and easier the alternative was, and the natural high is never quite the same as it used to be.

Imagine you're a child who just learned to ride a bicycle. It's now your favorite thing to do. You think about riding your bicycle all the time. If you never experience another mode of transportation, other than walking, you might never lose that feeling. Now you're a teenager and you get an electric scooter or a dirt bike. Your bicycle is still cool, just not as cool as your new toy. A few years later you get yourself a brand-new Harley Davidson. You can jump from zero to sixty as fast as you can shift the gears. The bicycle is still okay, the dirt bike can be fun, but when you've got the throttle pinned back and the wind in your face on that Harley there is nothing that can compare. Now, when you go for a bike ride you dream of your motorcycle. While the bike is still fun, the level of excitement you felt when you first learned to ride it never fully returns.

In *Opium for the Masses*, writer Jim Hogshire claims that Opium withdrawal is "no worse than a nasty case of the flu," and goes on to say that relapse is because "for many people, life is simply better with Opium than without it." While I have the utmost respect for the author, and his personal experience may have been accurately described in his work, I've lived a life that had me running with a circle of true addicts and my observations and experiences were contradictory to that of his. In my experience, *psychological addiction* is physical. You don't feel it in your muscles or stomach. It gnaws away at your mind. The chemical imbalance in the brain screams to be rectified. It's not your flawed personality, but your brain working against you to get what it desires.

Picture a man lost at sea. He runs out of food, then water. As dehydration sets in, he looks to the ocean to quench his thirst. The man is wise. He knows that he cannot drink the salt water of the sea. He knows that the body will use more water than he's taking in to get rid of all the salt and, thus, kill him by dehydration even faster. He suffers through thirst, dry skin and lips, and headaches. His muscles begin to cramp and fatigue sets in. Still, he knows he cannot drink from the ocean. The thirst becomes so strong that logic is discarded, and he goes against everything he knows thinking *I'll just have a sip*. One sip turns into two and before he realizes what he's doing he's gulping down mouthfuls of what he is craving. Before long, the man dies.

Once upon a time, I had a friend named Jake. He was a rather intelligent and empathetic man. He had an uncanny ability to listen to someone's problems and give sound advice that, after hearing, they would realize was the obvious solution. He was a problem solver. He became addicted to Opiates. It wasn't because he didn't understand addiction or that his life was unbearable. It was because he liked the euphoria that they provided. At first, it was an occasional good time. Soon it became an everyday want. Not long after that, it was a need.

One night, Jake decided he was going to stock up on pills from a little pharmacy he knew of in a strip mall in the ghetto town that I grew up in. He waited until all the stores were closed and climbed onto the roof of the building. He found an air conditioning duct and slipped through it into the store below. The problem, he soon found, was that the duct led into the wrong store. Not wanting it to be a wasted mission, he punched his way through the dividing wall and into the next store, and then the next, until he was finally in the pharmacy.

To ensure that he could escape, he pushed open the back door to verify that he wasn't now locked in. He found the pills he was looking for and immediately took a half dozen or so before continuing his raid. With plenty of time until sunrise, he nodded out on the floor of the pharmacy. What Jake didn't realize was that he set off a silent alarm when he tested the exit door. He awakened, still on the pharmacy floor with pills all around him, as the police entered. He tried to run but didn't get as far as the door. Jake was not a stupid man, yet the voice of addiction was yelling louder in his ear than the voices of logic and reason ever could. I'll never forget where I was the day that I got the call telling me that

Jake had overdosed. It was three years after the arrest that we jokingly referred to as the Drugstore Cowboy incident.

Dependence sets in quickly and at a slow pace. It tricks you into thinking it's not happening while slowly strengthening its hold on your mind. Opium, and opiates, will make you deceive yourself. By telling you that they are no more addictive than coffee or cigarettes, a bit of a half-truth, I could give you a false sense of confidence in approaching the subject. I don't believe that anyone has ever shit themselves when not being able to obtain a cigarette or projectile vomited from not having a cup of coffee. Those addictions are very real and have their own consequences, like headaches and an unrelenting longing, but neither produces the same consequence of missing an opiate fix when you can't satisfy the desire.

According to JohnsHopkinsMedical.org it only "takes a couple of weeks to become physically dependent on an Opioid." But physical addiction is not where dependence begins. The first stage of dependence, like love at first sight, can begin to take hold while you're high for the first time, especially if you don't believe it can. If all you're worried about is something that won't happen for weeks, why would you not partake in all the Opium you want all day every day for, say, a week or so? Or just all day every day for a long weekend? Then when it's time to go back to normal, surprise! You don't want to. That's because you're now chemically dependent. Control of your thoughts and desires falls by the wayside when it's easier to push back logic and rationalize your desires over your true needs.

People kill in the name of love. They can screw over close friends. They lie, cheat, and scam. Lives have been lost and relationships destroyed by the following of the heart. Without the right appreciation and control, opium can, and will, do the same. Remember the drug dealer's philosophy. On the first day, I'm your friend. On the second, I'm your best friend. By the third day, I'm your dealer. And while chemical addiction can be instantaneous, physical addiction comes relatively soon after. The only way to potentially avoid this is to follow the rules.

CHAPTER 6

THE RULES

The Rules

*Caution; Opioid. Risk of Overdose and Addiction. Ask
your healthcare professional if you should have Naloxone
on hand in case of overdose.*

Not many have outsmarted her their first time around and very few
can do so forever. The only rule that is guaranteed to keep you
alive and off the corner hustling your ass for a fix is simple. Do not
ingest opium or any of its derivatives. Most of us are generally
well-balanced, chemically, and the body's natural highs are quite
enough to keep us motivated and happy. Once you begin to mess
with that chemical balance, experiencing life without exogenous
alkaloids can be somewhat less fulfilling. If you stick to the opiates
your brain makes for you for free, you'll have a much better chance

of surviving this chaotic wasteland that we have inherited. It's so easy that you don't even have to think about it. I spent many years just saying no as friends and acquaintances offered me a bump here or a pill there. On an occasion or two, I tried Heroin and knew immediately that I should stay away. It was so powerful. Blissful. I didn't even mind projectile vomiting and scratching my arms raw, as long as she let me revel in my abandon.

While Morphine was the deadliest drug for nearly three-quarters of a century, pharmacology has caught up to Nature and surpassed her by miles. As mentioned earlier, a few grains of Fentanyl can kill an otherwise healthy adult man. The worst part of this reckless invention is that dealers are putting it not only in Heroin but in Cocaine and other desirable substances in order to make them more addictive. They're even putting them in bootlegged pills like Xanax and other opioids and it's impossible to tell the difference between the faux version with the snuck-in fentanyl, and the real thing. This has the added horror of people overdosing on things that otherwise do not cause death. Xanax, without alcohol or other drugs, does not cause death upon overdose. Only sleep, and lots of it. But Xanax laced with Fentanyl will kill you dead, if you take more than the dealer expected or if the dubious pusher fucked up and miscalculated the amount needed for a particular batch. Remember, Fentanyl is 200 times stronger than Morphine. It only takes a few specs the size of a grain of sand to kill.

Rule number one - Know your dose

Let me start by saying that the only reason for using Opium should be to relieve pain, a pain that your doctor has already prescribed opioid medications. I believe that natural medicines are less destructive to the body than pharmaceuticals. Opium should never be used as a recreational substance due to its highly addictive properties and potential for overdose. That said, if you are going to use any opiate, Opium is the healthiest and least harmful.

The rules are simple and yet somehow the most complicated to follow. First and foremost is to know your own dose. The main reason addicts die is overdose. The only acceptable method of experimenting with any psychoactive substance is to start with less than the dose it takes to feel an effect, systematically increasing the dose (after waiting an hour or so for each increment to hit) until the desired effect is achieved. Once that feeling is achieved, the dose must not be exceeded. The problem with this is that the body builds a tolerance to opium by decreasing the quantity of natural endorphins that are created. This creates a need for more of the substance to achieve the same effect and, over time, can cause one to lose interest in other pleasure-related activities. If you are building a tolerance, your use of opiates is already past the point of simple recreation.

There are several mistakes the user makes in this process. The first is to overestimate the dose needed to get high, either because of inexperience or because of the differences in the purity of the product being ingested. Unless you get your stash from a pharmacy, there is a high probability that your alkaloid levels and product purity vary from batch to batch. This includes the purity of Opium that you may either obtain from an outside source or process yourself from home-grown P. Somniferum. While Opium is far less deadly than other opiates, it does have a significant range of alkaloid density. Unadulterated air-dried Opium can contain between 8% and 20% Morphine. That means the purity can be more than double between batches.

Another reason for overdose is the impurity of the substance ingested. As mentioned earlier, opiates and other substances can be laced with chemicals that are far more deadly than what one thinks they are taking. Greed causes disreputable clandestine manufacturers to hide more addictive substances in their products in order to ensure their future slaves come back for more. This is the main reason I advocate for homegrown highs. If you can grow your own alkaloids, you know what's in the potion you are taking. If you must get high, use your own supply. All it takes is one shady manufacturer and countless lives are lost.

Other times, users also do their own mixing. While the mixing of any two substances can have adverse effects, some are much deadlier than others. Cocaine is a popular substance to do with opiates. Known as a speedball, each counteracts the side effects of the other creating a euphoria unlike any other, the downside being a much higher likelihood of death. The right amount of heroin can ease the anxiety of the cocaine and help the user come down more easily. The right amount of cocaine can help the heroin user stay awake through his high, instead of wasting it while asleep from the drug. But someone on cocaine needs more heroin to get high than he does when he uses the H alone, and vice versa.

By suppressing the negative side effects of each substance, the user thinks they can handle more, adding one or the other (and sometimes both) to achieve the desired high. When the coke wears off faster than expected, respiratory failure from the heroin causes overdose. When the H wears off before the Coke, a heart attack sneaks in. Even when done right, cocaine causes the body to use more oxygen while opiates slow breathing rates thus significantly increasing the risk of fatal respiratory failure. In the rock band Guns N' Roses alone, drummer Steven Adler had a stroke from speedballing that left him with a permanent speech impediment and guitarist Slash's heart stopped for eight minutes after doing the same concoction.

Still, the most common reason an *experienced* addict overdoses is miscalculation due to sobriety. Yup. Getting sober can be deadly to an addict if he or she relapses. Just as one's tolerance goes up with increased use, tolerance also gets lower after long periods of abstinence. Someone who's shooting fifteen bags of dope a day can tolerate that much without a problem, as long as the batches aren't laced and are of similar purity. Then they decide to change their life around. They miss all of the people they left behind while chasing their addiction, so they check themselves into rehab. After ten torturous days of detox, followed by a couple more weeks inside to make sure it sticks, they head out to face their new lives.

After a couple of days of being back in the unsanitized world of the living, they remember their apathy for the monotony of the day-to-day. As much as they want all of the benefits of sobriety, they long for the excitement that their old rituals (and a spike of euphoria) brought to the table. Even the act of copping drugs was a high in and of itself. Working, doing the dishes, and doing laundry can never compare to life on the streets and the rush of adrenaline that the dangers of addiction bring. Add to that missing the feeling of the alkaloid itself and you have a recipe for relapse that's hard to avoid. Just a taste is all they want. One little taste. So, they put the same two bags that used to bring such a small buzz into a spoon, add a little water, and suck it through a cigarette filter into a syringe.

As they push the needle in, slowly depressing the plunger on the syringe, they never get the chance to realize that what used to give them a slight buzz is now enough to cause respiratory depression. That's when pulmonary edema begins. Fluids begin to fill the air spaces in the lungs, causing foaming at the mouth and nose. Because opiates cause a suppression of the gag reflex, they begin to choke on the fluids and aspirate, the lungs filling with vomit. What the newly sober addict didn't consider was that the two bags that used to give him that slight buzz was now enough to take their life without them even knowing it. And you don't have to shoot heroin to overdose. Any opiate, including those in Opium, can cause death by whatever means it is ingested. If you don't know your dose, you're dead.

Rule two - Watch your habits

No single psychoactive substance should be taken every day. A good trick to enjoy nature's finest medicines without the annoyance of an addiction is to spread them out over the course of your week. While you may take a different psychoactive each day, no one substance should be taken too often. Mixing it up is not only good for keeping tolerance at bay and lowering the chance of addiction, but also a great way to keep from falling into patterns that become monotonous. Maybe this week one could take a little Opium to motivate yourself on Friday, then they might eat some Magic Mushrooms for a Saturday trip, ending the weekend by smoking some good old Cannabis on Sunday to relax while watching some movies. The following week the order can be rearranged, or the Shrooms may be exchanged for some Peyote or other psychedelic.

Periods of time should also be allowed for when no substances are consumed, allowing the brain to keep its normal regulatory function. Even something as innocent as Cannabis, if used every day, can cause irritability and, in extreme cases, absolute madness. I knew several people who smoked weed so much every day that when they had none, they became prone to verbally attacking those they loved as if their victims were their worst enemies. The venom that spewed from their lips was destructive to their relationships. One hit of weed and they were unaware of why they were mad to begin with. With opium, habitual use is much worse. The only highs that are nearly impossible to abuse are hallucinogens, like Acid and Mushrooms, due to the instantaneous tolerance they bring and the intensity of the high.

If you use opium daily for an extended period, you won't just be a dick, you'll need to use it every day for the foreseeable future in order to feel normal. Always remember that drug dealer's philosophy. By day three you are, on some level, addicted. After three days, a minor addiction might only manifest in simply explained ways. You might not sleep for hours after your normal bedtime because of what appears to be restless leg syndrome. Your thighs, calf muscles, and/or glutes begin to slightly ache, and the only cure is flexing them or a deep massage. While this may not seem like a big deal, it can cause sleep deprivation that leads to irritability and a generally dickish attitude. If use is continued on a regular basis, withdrawal symptoms will begin to manifest. Basically, you'll feel like you want to die. Nothing you believe in will stop you from going against all your values to get the dope boost you're looking for.

What I've found to be a maximum-use regimen is as follows: Once the perfect dose is found it cannot be exceeded. Don't use Opium more than twice a day. If you do, it will be harder to feel the same high while a single-use experience rarely requires an increase in dosage. Allow a minimum of several days between individual days of use. This will keep your tolerance at bay and avoid any chance of physical symptoms. If for any reason you may have decided to use Opium for multiple days, allow a minimum of ten days between any two or more consecutive days of doses. Never take opium three days in a row. If you do, you will likely experience some type of withdrawal. Finally, take a week off every couple of weeks to get yourself right in the head. This will help you to remember your core values and keep the brain fog (Opium's mind-control) that leads to bad choices at bay. For me, that was the difference between addiction and responsible use. Individual results will vary, as will dosage.

If you find yourself questioning the rules, remember that that's just the trick the mind plays in order to get what it craves. A slip here or there is not the end of the world until it is literally the end of your world. Questioning the rules is one thing. If you find yourself breaking them, you're already heading down a path that you may never be able to steer yourself away from. A good way to test your level of addiction is to follow the rules. If you can adhere to them without any trouble, you're likely winning the battle with addiction. The day you think you don't need the rules is the day you need them the most. If you can't take that week off, especially if you blow it off with the old line "I could take a week off - I just don't want to," you're in deeper than you think and should probably take a month or two to get your head straight.

CHAPTER 7
GET POPPIES

Where to get Papaver Somniferum

Buying Poppies

The quickest way to obtain Opium poppies is to buy them
wherever Poppies are sold. Many garden stores throughout the
United States carry potted Poppy plants. The problem with this
method is twofold. Florists and garden shops sell Papaver
Somniferum seasonally, so they are not always readily available
for use. Secondly, you must wait patiently for up to three months
for the bulbs to grow and ripen. If you're going to go through all of
that, you may as well grow them yourselves as I have outlined later
in this work.

There was a time in the not-so-distant past when most garden
stores carried and sold the dried bulbs of Papaver Somniferum for

ornamental purposes. That changed shortly after the publishing of Jim Hogshire's 1994 book, *Opium for the Masses: A Practical Guide to Growing Poppies and Making Opium*. There weren't many eyes on flower shops as sources of Opium prior to the book's widespread following. At least not in the eyes of the government and the law. Still, while Mr. Hogshire's book may have put the law's eyes on locally sourced Papaver Somniferum, as well as his own life, information should never be suppressed in an attempt to keep these gifts a secret. The more information out there, the more light we can shine on the absurdity of illegal vegetation. Hiding in the shadows causes misinformation and allows propaganda, like that put out by the government in the early twentieth century in the form of PSAs, to fool the population into supporting more anti-plant laws. Besides, the psychoactive plant revolution has already begun. They can't un-ring the bell.

Due to the ever-increasing popularity of opiates, their potential for abuse, and a wealth of information that now makes Opium available to anyone, finding ornamental dried Poppy pods in a garden store is rare. It's much easier for a quick internet search to provide sources outside of our normal range. Even these sources can be expensive and potentially a scam. If you order something that you're not supposed to buy, who are you going to complain to when you don't get it? That's why the easiest answer to obtaining all of the psychoactive plants your heart desires, and to ensure the survival of these plant species is to grow your own.

Obtaining Seeds

You can get Papaver Somniferum seeds at your local garden store or home store every spring. They are sold in small packets with names like Lauren's Grape, Bread Seed Poppies, Common Poppy, Black Swans, Swan's Down, Lilac Pompom, and more. You can find many different styles and colors to beautify your garden and enrich your botanical experience, yet if what you are looking for is *high* alkaloid content there is only one place you need to go. The supermarket.

Papaver Somniferum is grown to produce three main product categories. In 2020, Afghanistan alone produced 8.3 thousand tons of Opium Poppy. From there it is split into several raw materials. Natural opiates such as Morphine and Codeine are isolated from the raw opium in addition to Thebaine and Oripavine, the latter two being used by pharmaceutical companies to synthesize other opiates such as Hydrocodone and Oxycodone. The poppy straw is also used to harvest the remaining alkaloids. But waste not, the seeds of these intoxicating plants are not thrown to the birds. Those not used for replanting are packaged and shipped around the world for anyone and everyone who wants them, much like Opium used to be.

They can be found on your bagels and hard rolls, baked into breads and pastries, even in cookies. They are an excellent source of fatty oil that can be used for cooking, or as an ingredient in salad dressing. They add a nutty flavor and texture to baked goods. In Indian cuisine, they are even used in making curry. They're rich in fiber, essential Omega-6 fatty acids, calcium, copper, iron, manganese, magnesium, potassium, phosphorus, thiamine, and zinc and are a good source of protein. Head down the spice aisle of your favorite supermarket and you can even buy them in bulk. Even easier, the best way to get your hands on Papaver Somniferum seeds starts after you grow your first crop. Each ripe capsule contains hundreds of seeds that have an awesome germination rate. In the right conditions, you can just throw them across the garden floor and wait.

Home Grown Opium Poppies

Papaver Somniferum has an approximate growth cycle of 120 days and thrives in a temperate climate with low humidity and little rainfall. The seeds germinate easily and are well-established after the first month. It is a long-day plant, which means it won't produce flowers if it doesn't have at least twelve-hour days and does its best when planted a few of months before the summer solstice. There is little danger from insects or disease, so no fungicides and insecticides are necessary. When the pod is ripe, holes form around the crown and the wind shakes it like a rattle, blowing small amounts of seeds through the tiny holes until, eventually, it is empty. At this point, the cycle continues. For nature, it's that easy. For you, I've left a few pointers below.

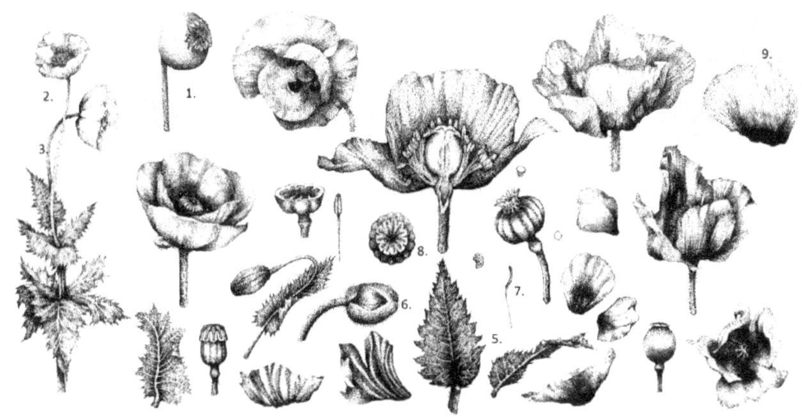

Papaver somniferum
Zharova Arsenia

Botanical Description

The basic parts of the Papaver Somniferum are as follows.

1. Seed pod or ovary
2. Peduncle or upper main stem
3. Tillers or secondary stems
4. Cotyledons or first leaves
5. True leaves
6. Sepals or the flower's protective cover
7. Anthers or pollen containing part of the plant
8. Stigma or pollen-receiving part of the plant
9. Petals

The Papaver Somniferum plant germinates quickly, appearing, as if out of nowhere, a few days after being sown. The first leaves, or cotyledons, are straight and almost grass-like in appearance. They are immediately followed by the first true leaves, which at first appear to be oval-shaped. It's not long before they become jagged-edged and start to look like miniature versions of their mature selves. If you've ever seen wild lettuce, Poppy leaves look quite similar. Next, sets of jagged leaf after jagged leaf will sprout with seemingly no end in sight. Just when you think it may be a weed, the peduncle will reveal itself, a phallic young bud hanging at its tip, its flower concealed beautifully by the sepals.

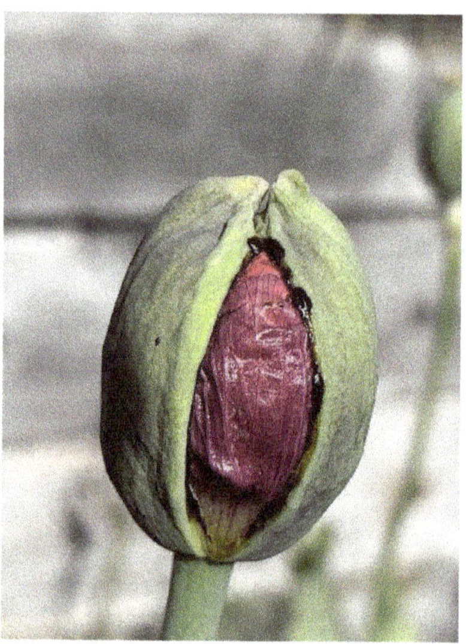

Sepals Parting (with an Opium seal)
Sandra Solanchick

No leaves will grow on the peduncle, while tillers, off-shoots of the main stem, may appear at intersections below the top set of leaves. If so, they will also have a flowering head at the tip. Each bud will become a seed pod, but the main head at the top of the peduncle will be the largest. Regardless of individual size, all will produce opium so, the more the merrier. As the flower begins to burst through the sepal, the petals appear. Pods hang like a question mark in what is known as the *hook stage*, slowly turning upward as the sepals fall, revealing the most beautiful of flowers. The flowers open to reveal petals of varying colors, from red to pale purple with a darker cuticle. Inside lies a ring of anthers surrounding the green ovary that boasts a crown of stigma.

In a matter of days, the flower becomes pollinated, and the leaves start to fall. The anthers drop next, leaving behind a beautiful ovary, the stigma lying gently around her tip. This is in no way the end of her journey. As the ovary expands, informing us that fertilization has taken place, the pod will swell as the seeds grow inside. The size increase can be astonishing the first time you witness it. When the crown of stigma, which starts out laying almost flat on top of the ovary, begins to rise up and the seed pod changes to a dull grey-green, Opium production is at its peak, and it is time to either score the plants or simply enjoy their beauty until they fully ripen and begin to disperse their seeds.

Germinating and care of seedlings

Papaver Somniferum seeds, also known as poppy seeds, are the same poppy seeds on your bagel or a good New York City hard roll. Germination of these seeds takes little, if any, practice. They are hardy seeds and will germinate quickly when they are introduced to moisture. Unlike other types of seeds which require the botanist to jump through various hoops, such as moistening them in paper towels or soaking them in order to have a high success rate, simply throwing Poppy seeds on the ground and keeping them moist will ensure an amazing germination rate of nearly 100%.

There are many who will tell you that store-bought poppy seeds are sterilized and will not germinate. Nothing could be further from the truth. In order to test their theory, I purchased several different brands of Poppy seeds in the spice isles of different supermarkets and grocery stores, simply tossing them in the garden. From that experience, I found that the germination of Papaver Somniferum from store-bought seeds is on par with that of freshly harvested seeds. Nearly all the seeds I have ever dropped have sprouted. Germination is the easy part. What comes next takes a little thought and talent. In California, the best time to start

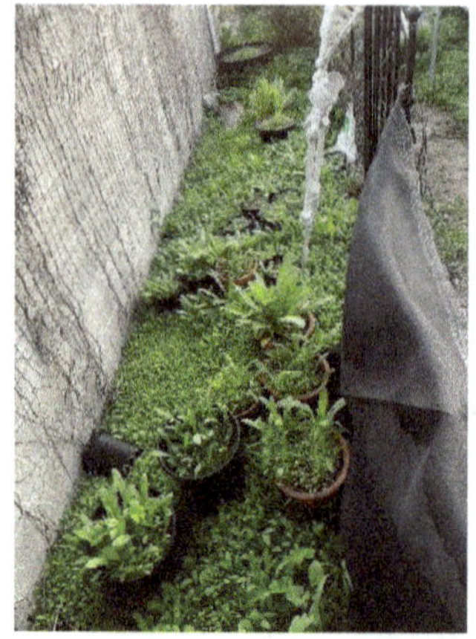
A blanket of newly germinated poppy seeds

Papaver seeds outdoors is from just after the winter solstice to mid and even late January.

The seedlings of the Papaver plant are delicate. This is the main reason we don't bother with multi-step germination tactics. Why go through all that trouble when you don't have to? As with anything, the simplest strategy that produces the best results is the correct way to do it. Other than being unnecessary, handling the seeds after germination is detrimental to their survival. The hairlike sprouts are fragile, and prone to destruction from transplanting, as well as from the elements. Wind and rain, even garden sprinklers, can rip them to shreds. I've walked away from a blanket of sprouts that resembled a healthy lawn only to find that after harsh weather, or powerful sprinklers that I forgot to turn off, only sporadic patches of seedlings were left hiding around rocks, garden ornaments, or other plants.

The best method of watering, when growing in pots, is bottom watering. Simply place the pots in water (in a sink or another container) keeping the water level lower than the top of the soil. This allows the water to enter the pot through the drainage holes as the soil soaks it up. When the top of the soil begins to show dampness, remove the pots from the water and allow them to drain before returning them to their usual location. Only water your plants when the soil is dry at a depth of one inch or about the distance from the tip of your index finger to your first knuckle.

When bottom watering is not possible, a drip system works well. If neither can be achieved, such as when the Papavers are planted directly in your garden's soil, just water gently. Hold the watering can as close to the surface of the soil as possible or set the hose on a low pressure. Be nice. Try not to beat them up too badly. When they reach a few inches tall there will be little need to worry about the normal forces of nature.

Watching and Waiting (but what about pests?)

Once the Poppies start to produce jagged leaves reminiscent of some lettuces, you no longer have to be worried about wind and rain. From here on out, only water once weekly. Poppies prefer loose, well-draining soil and don't need a lot of water once they have taken hold. There is no need to water more often and less is better if your soil retains any moisture. Again, I use the one-inch rule. If you poke your finger down an inch and feel *any* moisture, don't water. If it's dry, give it a little drink. It's been said that over-watering dilutes the opium content of the Poppy. I call bullshit on that, too. While over-watering anything can lead to stem rot, everything needs water. In all of my experiments, more water does little, if anything, to change the Opium content while underwatering can stunt growth. That said, Papaver needs less water than your average house or garden plant once it is established.

Now it's time to watch and wait. Poppies start out looking like weeds, jagged leaf after jagged leaf spiraling out from the center for several weeks with seemingly no end in sight. Then, just when you start to forget about looking for it every day, a single stem carrying a small bulb, its head hung low and limp, emerges. Slowly over the next several days, the pod begins to lift itself towards the sun. Just before it becomes fully erect, the two sepals begin to part revealing the pedals. Sometimes the petals are a brilliant red but most are a pale purple with a ring that is a few shades darker, reminiscent of the cuticle of a fingernail, closer to the bulb.

While this is the common shade, the type you will almost certainly get from the spice isle of the grocer, many different variations exist ranging in colors from almost a black purple to nearly white, and every shade in between. There are also different varieties of leaves. Most have four flat leaves of an almost rounded triangular shape that together create a circle around the bulb, the darker inner cuticle adding four darkened spots to the design, while others can have a double set of crunched-up leaves that look similar to that of a carnation. Still others have jagged leaves that resemble a frayed flag that has been left to the wind for too long. You can find the seeds for these online or for sale at any nursery or home store. There is no end to the beauty of this plant, or to its diversity.

Rodents, as well as other animals, love to eat your poppies. Junkie rats are the biggest problem you will discover. I had a garden of Papaver that was planted at the most optimal time. Sets of jagged leaves reached two or more feet in height before they started to reveal their peduncle. Just as the bulbs began to form, junkie rats ate every pod before I even got to see them. All that was left were stems with a small amount of Opium sealing the wounds left at the site of their decapitation. Each day a new plant had the tell-tale brownish latex where the ovaries should have been. The entire crop was lost to these drug-addicted rodents.

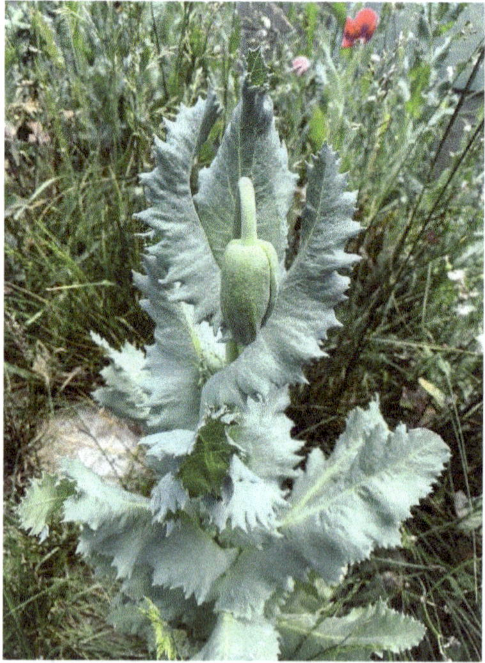

Angel of Death

Indoor growing

The only difference between indoor and outdoor growing is that you have to control the light hours when growing indoors. Many of the plant species that I have grown indoors require long light hours during vegetative growth followed by shorter hours to stimulate sexual maturity, budding, and seed growth. Papaver Somniferum is quite the opposite. She is a long-day plant, meaning that she requires the light hours to increase to stimulate budding. Unlike Cannabis, which I like to grow in an 18-hour day cycle during vegetation followed by a 12-hour day/night cycle to stimulate budding, Poppies can be vegetative in the 12/12 photoperiod. When they reach an optimal size, an increase in light hours to 18, followed by 6 hours of night, signals the plant that it is time to push up the peduncle.

Harvesting

After the sepals drop, you can relax and enjoy the beauty of the flowers for a few days at which point the wind, or simply gravity, robs her of her petals. If you can retrieve them from your garden before they are lost, they are excellent for pressing in a book or wrapping your homemade Opium in for storage. At this point, the Poppy pod will begin to look like those depicted in most reference pictures. It may be thin, and egg-shaped, or larger and almost round. The ovary will continue to swell and will eventually range in size from that of a marble to the size of a child's closed fist, the largest being too big to wrap your hand around.

The stigma of the Poppy is the easiest way to determine when to harvest Opium. While the stigma of the Opium Poppy can refer to the mark of disgrace associated with her use, in this section we use stigma to refer to the part of the plant that receives pollen during fertilization. When the petals fall, giving free rein to the wind that will eventually steal the anthers as well, only the stigma remains on the pod. The stigma makes up the halo around the top of the ovary, or pod. At first, the stigma lay horizontal and flat, like a disk. As the ovary swells, the stigma begins to point upward. When they are nearly vertical, think of the fingers on a hand holding a cup from the bottom, then the Opium is ready for harvesting. The Poppy pod will also change color slightly, from bright green to a dull bluish green. Not all poppies in a garden will be ready at the same time. Pay close attention to each and harvest them individually when the time is right.

Scoring method

This is the method that has been used for millennia to extract the Poppy's latex, better known as Opium, and not much has changed since the invention of the blade. About two weeks after the petals have dropped, and the poppy pod looks ready for harvesting as mentioned above, the Poppy pods are scored with a knife at a depth of 1 to 1.5 millimeters. Specialized knives are made with multiple blades. This is run vertically over the pod in several areas to maximize the wounds. If the cuts are too shallow the latex will coagulate too soon and heal the wounds, with little Opium obtained. If they are too deep, the Opium will drip back into the pod and stop the lactifers from producing.

When done properly, the latex will slowly ooze from the wound, coagulating on the surface of the pod. The next day, the latex is scraped off and collected to be dried further. An average of 80 milligrams of Opium per pod is the approximate yield. The raw Opium, containing a high percentage of water, is then allowed to dry until it is the consistency of a putty. From there, it can be smoked, eaten, or processed further by dissolving it in water and filtering it to remove plant matter. It is, again, dried to the consistency of dough. The more matter that is removed by this method, the purer the Opium will be. Over hundreds of years, this process has been refined to maximize yield and potency, depending on its intended use.

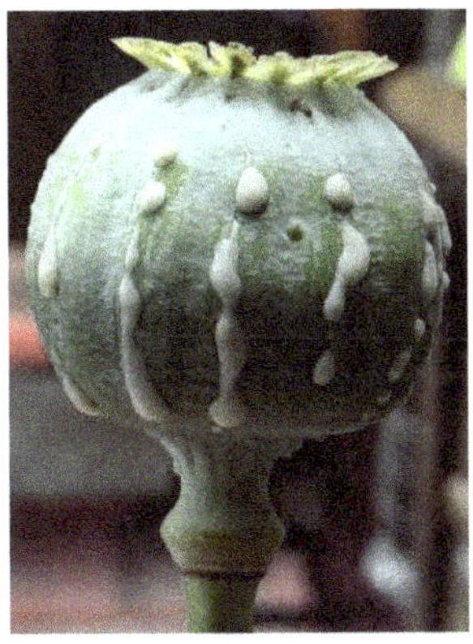

Score method

Pin method

Another way to harvest the latex is to poke the pod at a depth of 1 to 1.5 millimeters with a sharp object, such as a quill, pin, or wire. I've even heard of people using the bottom string of a guitar. While this is extremely time-consuming, it's a decent method for someone who has a small-scale, personal use operation where they have a small crop and want a maximum yield. A tool can be made that pokes dozens of holes simultaneously at the perfect depth. The key to maximizing this method is to prick the flesh of the ovary every sixteenth of an inch for a total of 289 jabs per square inch, or over 3000 holes leaking Opium.

The upside to this method is that, if done right with a properly fabricated tool, you avoid cutting too deep, causing the Opium to be lost in the pod or to spill onto the ground. The downside is that it can only be done successfully one time per pod. Again, for the home grower, and for personal use, this is usually enough. The healed pod can then be dried to make tea which can be further reduced as described in the *raw opium straw extract* model.

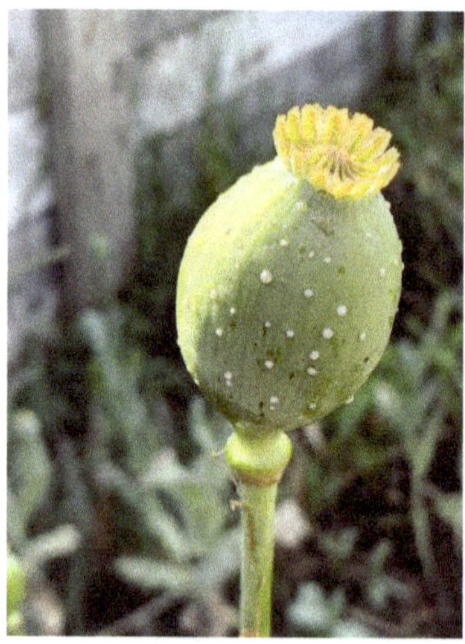

Pin Method

Let it be

Another way of harvesting a form of Opium from the Papaver Somniferum is to just let it finish its life cycle. I prefer this method for many reasons, the first being ease. As I mentioned earlier, the proper way to do anything is the easiest way in which the best results are obtained. The easiest way to get usable Opium is to simply do a water extraction from the dried Poppy pods. This is known as Poppy Straw extraction, Poppy Straw being the dried parts of the Papaver Somniferum. There is nothing simpler than letting the plant complete its life cycle. On the small scale of personal use, there is little to nothing gained by milking the pod prior to the *raw Opium extraction from Poppy straw*, outlined below.

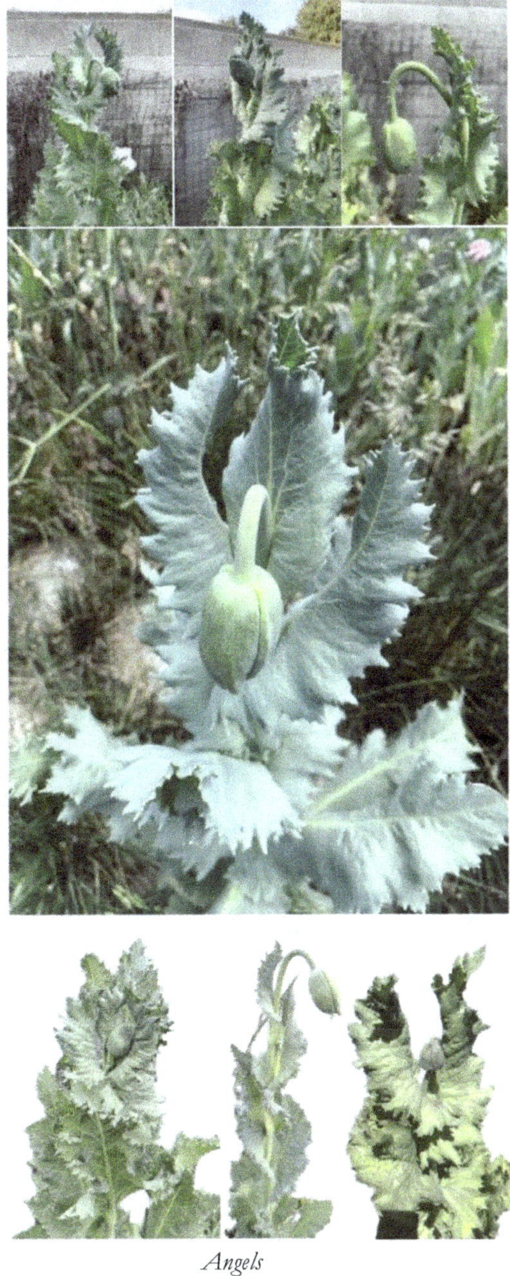

Angels

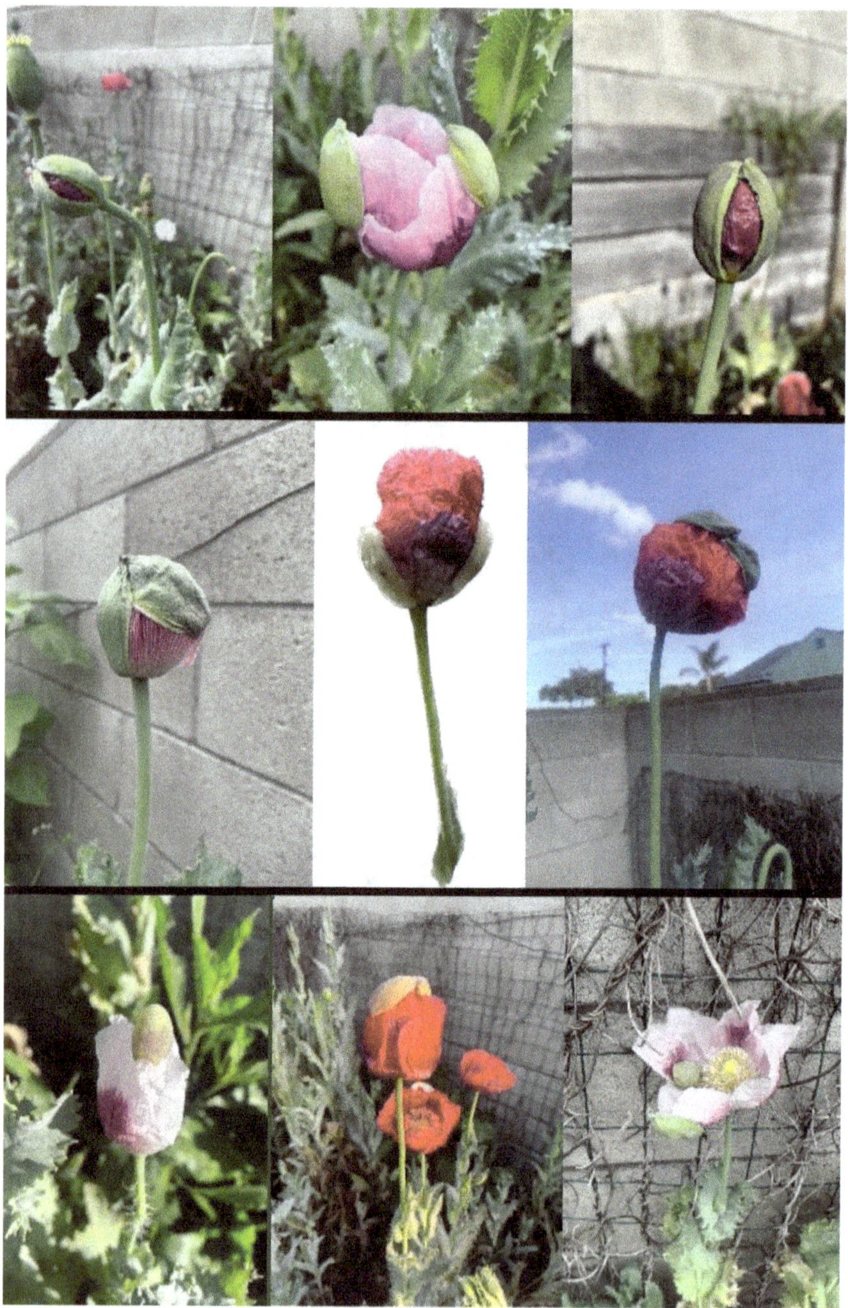

Sepals

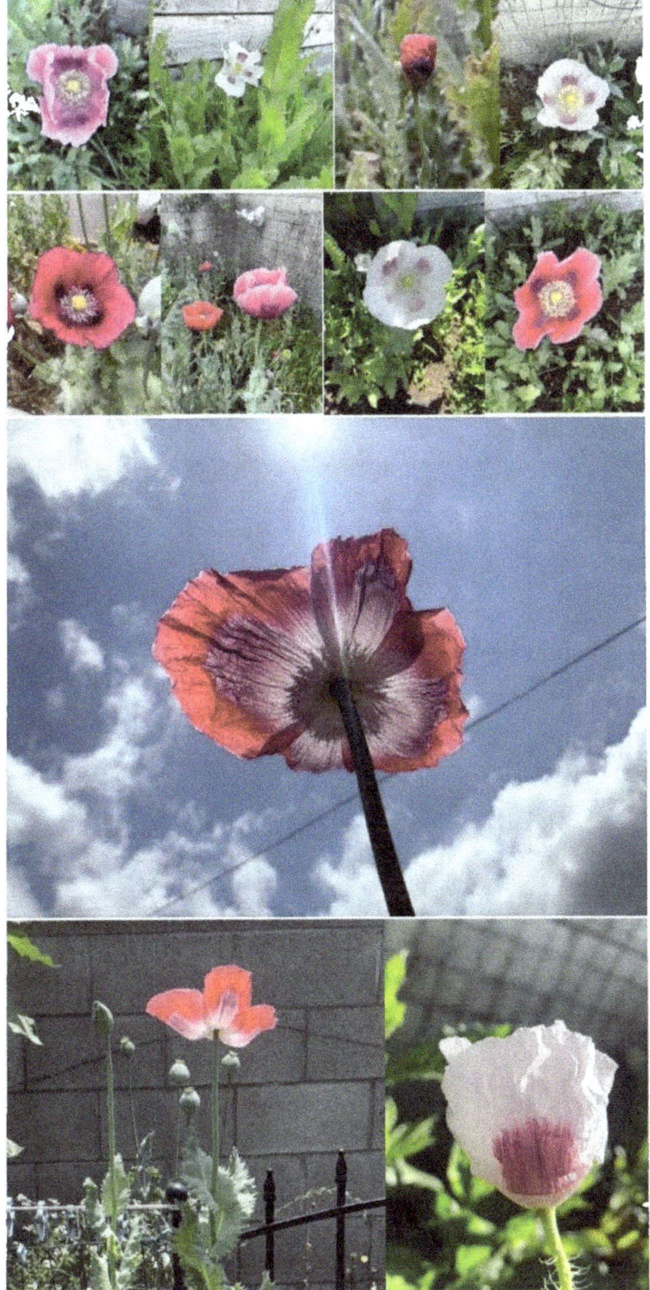

Flowers

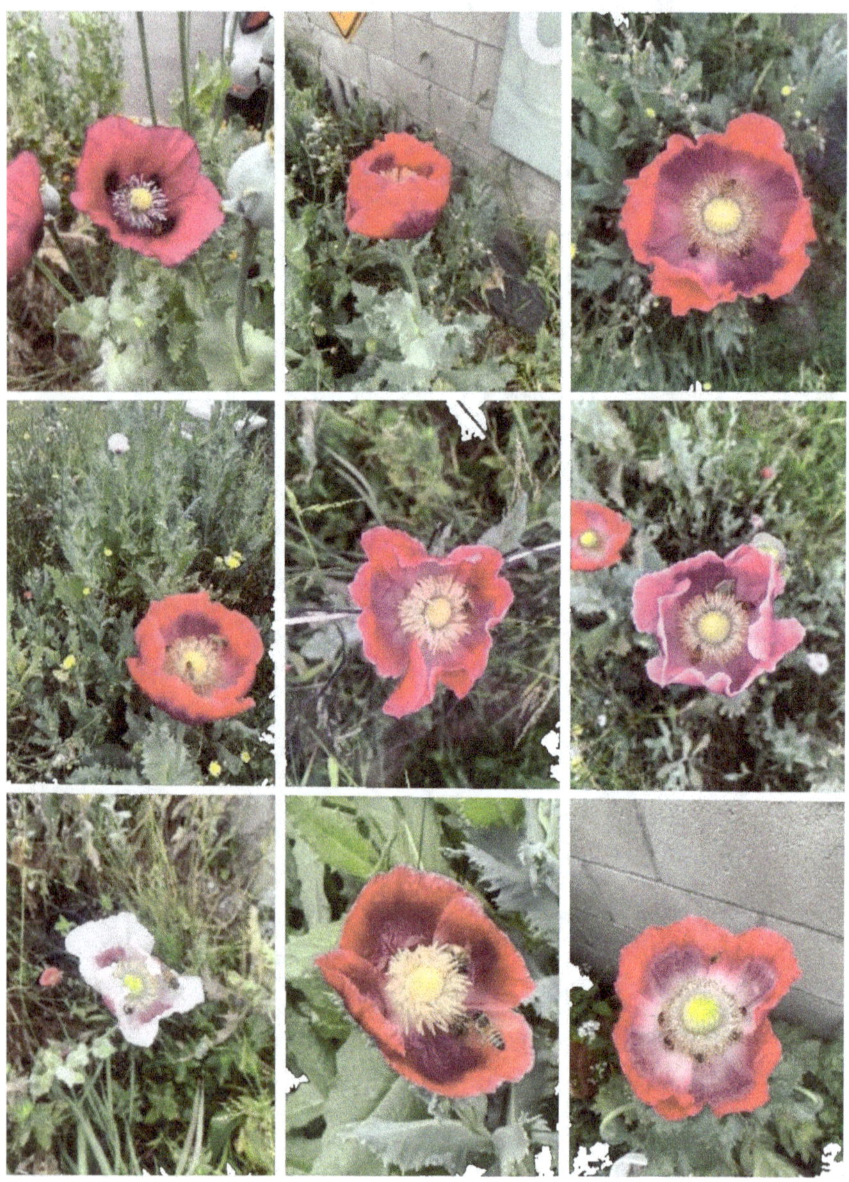

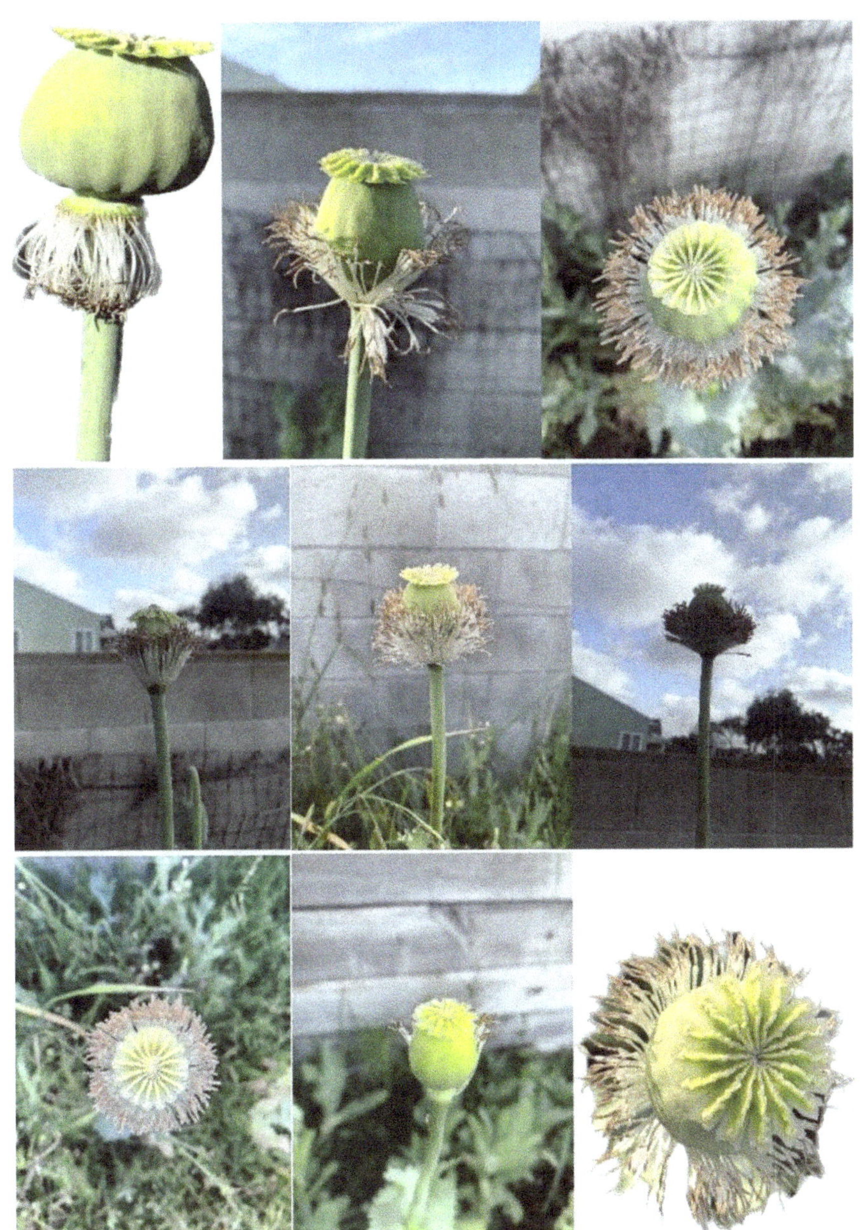

Anthers

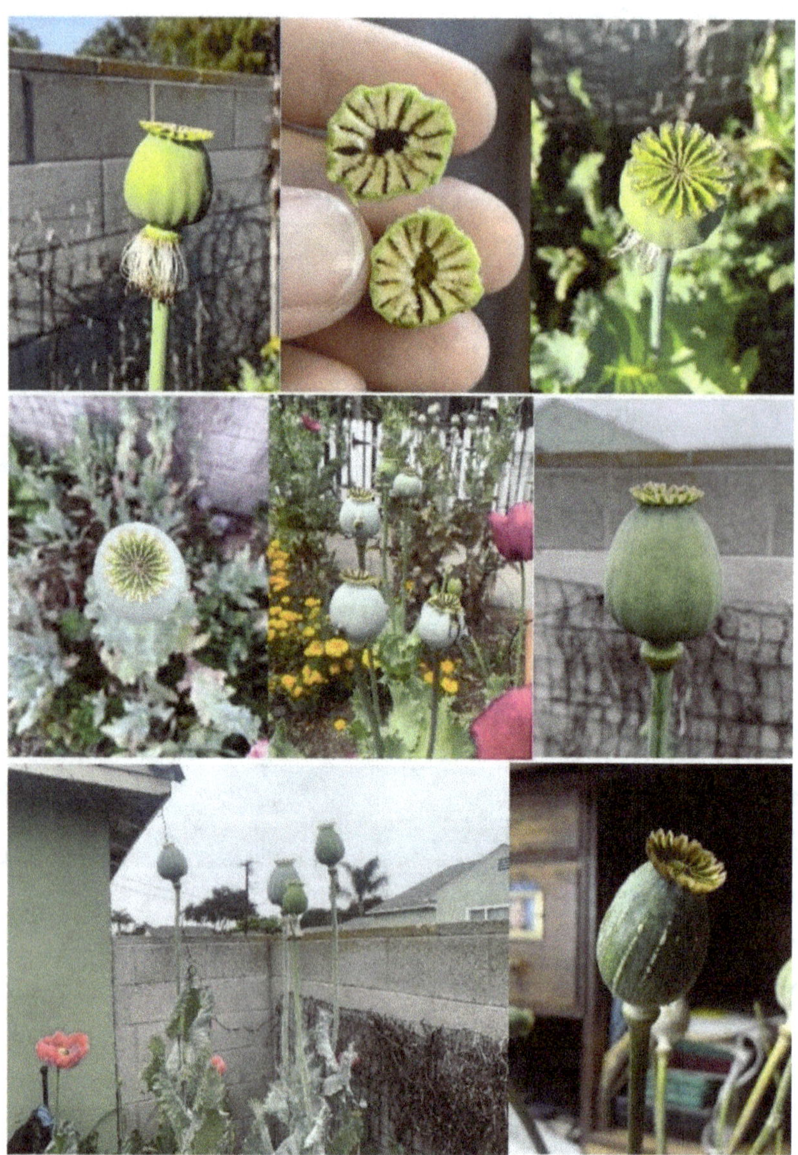

Pods

CHAPTER 8

MAKE TEA

Making your own Opium

The United States Government has instructions for the manufacture of Morphine and Heroin on their website, NCJRS.gov. I have heard the National Criminal Justice Reference Service referred to as the National Criminal and Junkie Reference Service. They have publications available to the general public that provide detailed step-by-step instructions for cultivating, extracting, and processing Opium first to Morphine and then to Heroin. They also have a publication with similar instructions on the process of cultivating and extracting pure cocaine from the leaves of the Coca plant. Feel free to look these publications up if you want to. I can't responsibly repeat those instructions here, but I will give you the gist of it later on. The processes described herein are for informational purposes only and are purely hypothetical.

In my personal opinion, all you need is Opium. Why fuck with nature's most powerful medicine? It has all the benefits and allures of the derivatives without the concentrated strength that so easily kills the user. When one enjoys a fine wine, they don't usually distill it to obtain pure ethanol. That would defeat the purpose of making the wine to begin with. Why, then, separate and concentrate any of the Opium alkaloids? All you need to do to obtain all the painkilling and mood-elevating properties of the Opium Poppy is as follows.

Poppy Tea (aka EZT)

The potions of Witches, Sorcerers, Shaman, and snake oil salesmen were but simple extractions of alkaloids, and other useful ingredients, from plants. These early medicine men and women knew that certain plants had magical healing powers, a knowledge our society has all but forgotten. For as long as humans have had the ability to write, they wrote first of the *magical* concoctions that both healed physical pain and transported them to a reality that differed from our own. The oldest potion of record is that of a concoction containing Opium that dates back over 5,000 years. The word potion comes from the Latin potus, or to drink, which later evolved into potionum, while the Ancient Greeks used the same word for potion as they did for medicines, pharmaka.

While the word pharmaceutical is quite obviously derived from this, pharmaceuticals are rarely potions anymore. They now rely solely on what is thought to be the active ingredient of a single source material, rather than a multi-source cocktail. While this has the benefit of prescribing a regulated dose of whichever alkaloid we prefer, it is at the detriment of the natural mixtures which may well be the key to unlocking their potential. By far the oldest way to relieve pain, and elevate the spirit as well, was to drink the tea of the Poppy.

Opium tea is made by simply crushing and bringing two to five poppy pods, about 10 grams of Papaver Somniferum bulbs from which the seeds have been removed, almost to a simmer in two cups of water. Let it sit in the hot water for 15 to 25 minutes. The effects are long-lasting, from four to six hours, and the pods can be re-boiled with enough alkaloids left in them for a second cup to be enjoyed. Each large poppy pod provides approximately one dose per person, per cup, with each subsequent extraction being about half as potent as the previous. Dosages vary based on the size of the poppy bulb and the concentration of opium per pod. One poppy the size of a lime (per cup, per person) was a good starter dose for me and I'm 6 feet tall and 200 pounds. As with anything one has never done before, care should be taken to start out with a smaller dose and wait one hour to see what the effects (and side effects) are.

Dopium - Raw Opium extraction from Poppy straw

Opium extraction from dried opium poppy pods is a simple procedure. If someone has the basic skills it takes to make the tea described above, they can make this crude yet potent form of Opium. For millennia, humans have used two Opium extraction methods. The scoring and harvesting method mentioned previously, and the one I will detail below. Harvesting from live pods, while resulting in a superior product, is not completely necessary and will not result in a yield even close to that of the following process. Scoring and scraping also have the added complication of being laborious.

Scoring and harvesting is definitely a fun experience, yet it quickly becomes a chore when you realize the atomity of the yield. More than half of the world's Morphine comes from extraction from Poppy straw, which is the dried pods, leaves, and stems of the Papaver Somniferum. I advocate for the use of only the pods, when done on a scale as small as this, due to the higher concentration of alkaloids. You can use the leaves and stems separately, with a much weaker end result, if you wish.

The process is as follows: Grind up 18 poppy pods, with an average weight of 4-5 grams each after removing the seeds, in a blender. The reason for not using more pods is that water can only hold so much and, in my experiments with a 7-quart slow cooker, more than twenty pods slow-cooked twice does not yield any more of the end product. While water can hold 149mg of Morphine per liter, and almost five times that amount if the water is boiling, there's a lot more than Morphine in the water during this extraction. In this case, more is not better. It's a waste.

In a 7-quart slow cooker, maximum yield is achieved using between 64 and 80 grams of dried, crushed, and de-seeded Papaver Somniferum bulbs. I prefer to go with the lesser amount as the yield tends to plateau from there on up. More raw material can be used in a larger vessel and, likewise, less should be used in a smaller one. Less poppy straw in more water doesn't alter the results, however, too many heads in less water will result in less than the maximum final product. When done correctly, the yield is approximately 30% to 35% of the starting weight. The resulting material is neither completely dried and hardened nor sticky to the point of transference to one's fingers when kneaded like clay. 80 grams of heads yield about 25 to 28 grams of Dopium, 60 grams yield about 18 or so grams, and so on.

When grinding the bulbs, poppy straw doesn't have to be ground to a fine powder. The goal is to create the most surface area as possible to extract as much Opium as possible. The more surface area, in theory, the more Opium will be released. That said, I find little difference in quality and quantity using pieces the size of your fingernail versus fine powder, and splinters are easier to filter out than dust. For the sake of limiting steps, I usually just crush the dried bulbs in my hand, dumping out the seeds into a separate container as I go.

The crushed or ground pods are placed in a 6- or 7-quart slow cooker and submerged in as much water as the vessel will hold. The crockpot is set to low and allowed to do its job for twelve hours or more, and an additional 12 hours on warm being the recommended amount of time for maximum alkaloid extraction. You may read elsewhere that heat destroys the quality of the product by vaporizing or otherwise degrading the alkaloids. This is simply untrue. The United Nations Office on Drugs and Crime has a publication on its website called *Effect of Temperature on the*

Estimation of Morphine in Opium that outlines the degradation of Morphine based on heat. Without getting into too much detail, our process won't hurt the goodies.

Filter the liquid through a small strainer or a heavy dense cloth. A deep fryer filter wrapped in dense cloth works well. Still, I find cloth teabags to be optimal. When they have finished the first boil you can simply lift them out of the water and place them in a pot of fresh water for round two. The end goal is not to crystalize Morphine salts and make Heroin. In this scenario, the impurities that pass through the filter act as a filler for the end product much as the fillers they use in prescription pills. A 5mg hydrocodone pill is quite large, yet 5mg of powder is about the size of the tip of a ballpoint pen. The more concentrated an alkaloid concoction is, the more likely one is to take too much, or overdose.

After filtering, put the liquid in the refrigerator for later. Place the *tea* bag, or mass of poppy pulp left in the filter, back in the slow cooker, submerge in water, and repeat the 12-hour extraction. Filter again and discard the now leached plant material. You'll see that the liquid is much more translucent in the second round. That's because we got most of the *juice* in the first batch. The second batch is to catch whatever we may have missed due to the solubility of the alkaloids and other materials. Place the *tea* in the refrigerator to cool for several hours.

When the liquid has cooled to the temperature of the refrigerator, approximately 40 degrees Fahrenheit (4 degrees Celsius) it is removed and filtered through a fresh filter and a clean cloth in the same method outlined previously. This is known as cold-water extraction. Some of the plant material and other impurities that are soluble in hot water are less soluble in cold while the alkaloids in Opium remain dissolved at cooler temperatures. Because of this, cold-water extraction helps to purify the yield. I knew a doctor who would perform this extraction when taking opioid medications in order to remove the inert ingredients, not to increase potency but to purify the substance he was introducing to his system.

Next, we combine the liquid from both extractions, which is returned to the slow cooker for reduction. If all the liquid does not fit in the vessel you can begin to reduce the first batch, adding the second batch as water is evaporated and room in the vessel is created. Reduction is achieved by leaving the crockpot on the *warm* setting, allowing the low heat to aid in the evaporation process. I fluctuate between settings depending on my need for speed. As mentioned earlier, a slow cooker will not get hot enough to hurt the alkaloids. One might even leave it on high for a short period of time in order to speed the process, but only if someone is there to oversee the progress. We don't want a dry vessel. If the crockpot cracks, the experiment is ruined.

During the reduction process, which is simply heat-assisted evaporation, you will see residue precipitate around the water line. With a clean spray bottle full of pure water, the waterline is misted while being rubbed with a gloved finger to dissolve any precipitates back into the potion. I use the hot *tea* to help dissolve the solids, misting my finger to ensure it doesn't get burned in the process. The crockpot is hot, the liquid is hot. It's easy to leave the digit in too long and, ouch.

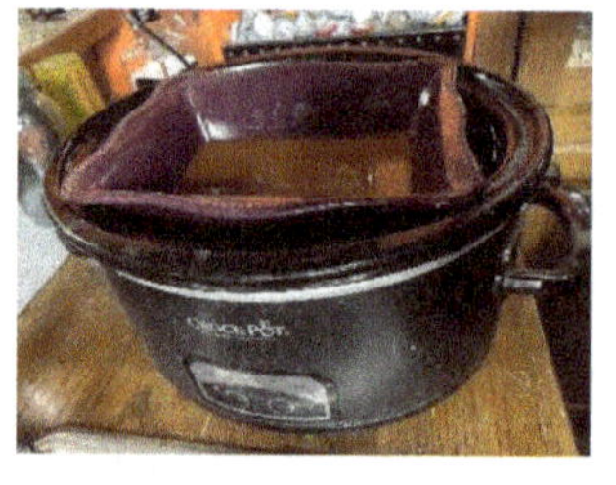

When the crude Opium extract is the consistency of a thick gravy, not quite solid but barely a flowing liquid, it is placed in a shallow Pyrex or ceramic vessel that fits into the crock pot, but whose edges are wider than the top of the crock pot, suspending it high above the slow cookers bottom. The slow cooker is then filled until the water touches the bottom of the second vessel. The crockpot is now set to high. Using a square ceramic baking dish allows the original crock pot lid to hold in heat while also allowing the water vapor rising out of the ceramic dish to condense on the lid, dripping down the sides and back into the water contained in the slow cooker below. This distillation has the added benefit of lessening the number of times you have to refill the crock pot due to the evaporation of the water in the lower chamber. Still, you must keep a close eye on the water level in the slow cooker. A crock pot is not meant to be used dry and will crack not long after all the water evaporates. Top it off whenever the water level falls below half.

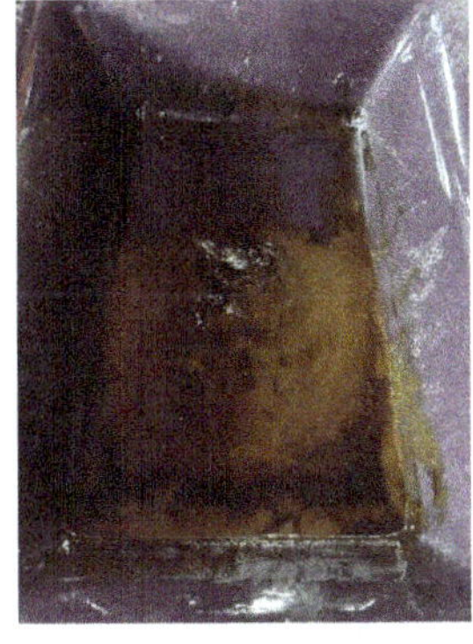

Once the liquid thickens to a sludge it is time to get to work. With a razor blade or some other heat-resistant squeegee, gather the viscous liquid into the center of the dish. A razor is effective in scraping the dried extract along the edges back into the sludge where it can rehydrate. At first, you will be pushing semi-solids to the center, while the more liquified parts flow back into the emptied space. Soon the whole mass will become a gooey paste, followed by the consistency of wet dough. For convenience's sake, you want to keep an eye out that you don't remove too much water, creating a hardened cake. If this happens, don't throw your product away. Water can be added to rehydrate, or you can always use it in a Laudanum recipe. The desired consistency is achieved when the dough no longer sticks to the tool or your fingers yet is still pliable.

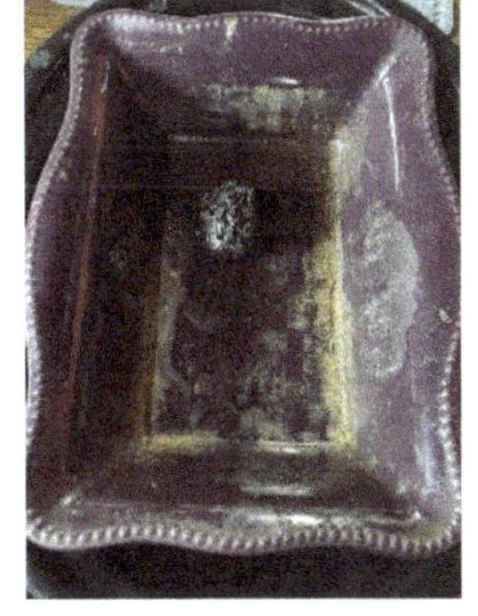

When the Opium is solid enough to be rolled in your hand without leaving more than a stain behind, but not so dry that it can't be manipulated like clay, it's time to make Opium balls. The crude Opium is kneaded in the hands, mixing the alkaloids within to provide an even distribution. At this point, it is rolled on a hard wooden surface, such as a cutting board, until it is the width of a pen. Chunks are broken off at a length equal to the width and rolled into balls that should weigh approximately 0.5 grams. If the opium is to be eaten in pill form, it can then be inserted into vegetarian or gelatin capsules. The sizes of these capsules grow smaller the higher the number. Size O (which holds about a gram to a gram and a half) or smaller is recommended, size 1 being about a half gram.

While Opium made by this method is not nearly as potent as purified true Opium, it only contains about a fifth of the Morphine as the true latex, it is still a very powerful and deadly concoction when not respected. One can easily feel the effects of a half gram of this sticky gum, as it can contain approximately 10mg of morphine, along with codeine and other alkaloids. As plants vary in their concentration, this amount can be more or less depending on many factors, including genetics, and growing conditions. For this very reason, Opium is not something that a true dosage can be recommended and, therefore, can be dangerous, if not deadly. This is also why the isolation of Morphine by our friend Friedrich Serturner was so important to the field of medicine. Prior to his discovery, Opium's use as an analgesic could either leave a patient in agony or dead.

Storage

Ways to store Opium have varied over the centuries. In 19th century India, for instance, Opium was kneaded and rolled into a 6-inch diameter sphere. In a bowl with a slightly larger diameter, Papaver petals were laid and coated with an inferior liquid Opium, known as lewah. Each petal overlapped the previous one, the lewah gluing them in place. The ball of Opium was placed inside, and the petals wrapped around it until the sphere was completely covered. The Opium ball, now completely sealed by lewah-soaked petals, was placed on a drying rack where it would be turned daily by young boys.

Storage of Opium doesn't have to be that complex. If one plans to put their Opium in capsules, no further steps are needed, and it can be kept indefinitely. Otherwise, a ball can be stored as mentioned above or simply placed in a silicone container. A wooden egg-like container was the preferred method of storage in the days of the

Opium dens of New York and San Francisco. For the most part, any container is fine if the Opium is dry enough not to stick to the inside. Further drying only causes the opium to become solid and hard to cut or break. Too much moisture can only make a mess. Sealing the containers is recommended as a particularly humid day can turn your perfect clay into wet tar.

Morphine and Heroin Production Summary

The Alkaloid isolation and conversion to Heroin I promised to summarize is also fairly easy, though I find no reason to bother attempting it for any purpose other than medical need. It begins by dissolving Opium in water. The liquid is then run through coffee filters until there are no solids left to be caught. Calcium hydroxide, or slaked lime, is added to precipitate non-morphine alkaloids. The liquid is again filtered and re-heated. Ammonium chloride is then added to adjust the PH to 8 or 9 and allowed to cool. In a couple of hours Morphine base, known by the Chinese name *pi-tzu*, precipitates out of the liquid and is caught in a filter. Some hydrochloric acid, activated charcoal, heat, filter, and voila. Morphine Hydrochloride.

The process for converting the Morphine to Heroin is just as easy and uses chemicals that are just as readily available. It's all just cooking with science. Before you go searching the government websites for the step-by-step instructions they've published, remember that Morphine extraction is highly illegal, in and of itself. Going further than making some tea is crossing a line that will likely land you in prison or dead. There's a fine line between personal use and criminal manufacture of a controlled substance with the intent to distribute. If someone else dies because of your little hobby, or if anyone dies while you're committing any crime, you're guilty of murder.

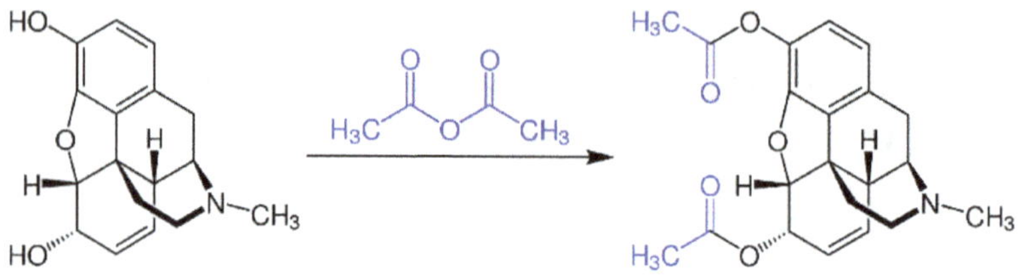

Heroin to Morphine

CHAPTER 9

METHODS OF INGESTION

Personal History (Part II)

I've lost many loved ones due to overdose, the survivors left chained to their addiction. I've never known anyone who could control their use of pharmaceutical opiates or heroin. The ones who have passed away all claimed to *know their dose*. I've known guys who maintained a fifteen-bag-a-day Heroin habit and others who died from doing just one or two. I've answered countless phone calls from their loved ones and placed dirt on the coffins of my brothers as all around me wept. I've woken to the cries of someone whom I consider a brother as he rose to find our young friend dead on my couch. They died from eating pharmaceutical opiates, from shooting Heroin, from snorting Heroin, or from snorting crushed-up pills.

The addicts that don't die live on the edge of heaven and hell, one mistaken dose or unknown contamination away from death. A man we will call Adam, one of my oldest friends and someone I've known for over 35 years, reached out to me recently to catch up.

His message read *[my son is] gonna be 29 years old. It's hard to believe [that] everyone said I would be the first to die out of all of our friends and all our friends are dead and I'm a grandpa. Life's a trip,* he continued, "*2 heart attacks and 14 overdoses and I'm still standing!!* He wears those statistics like a badge of honor and yet, under the surface, he wishes he could erase the drug from his memory.

Adam feels the damage of years of abuse. *Live fast, die young* was his motto. He never expected to reach his 30s, let alone his 50s. He never cared about what drugs did to his body because he didn't think he would make it long enough to feel the negative effects. Years of abuse have left him a shell of his former self. He's spent much of his life homeless on the streets of New York and his only regret is Heroin. His only wish is that he could kick the addiction and get back to his true love, Angel Dust. The end of his message read *I need to stop doing dope and get back to smoking dust,* and *I need to get off the dog food. If I don't have it, I'm sick as a dog.*

Whether she kills you fast or swallows your soul slowly while you remain shackled to her, Heroin and other pharmaceutical opioids always lead to death. I'm not sure which is worse. A lifetime of chasing your tail, without any hope of ever catching that perfect high again, or the quick end that many find all too soon. Either way, it's a waste of a life. I'm of the opinion that, without further purification, the road followed on the way to self-controlled use of Opium does not end so abruptly. The higher you go, and the more quickly you reach that height, the harder you will fall.

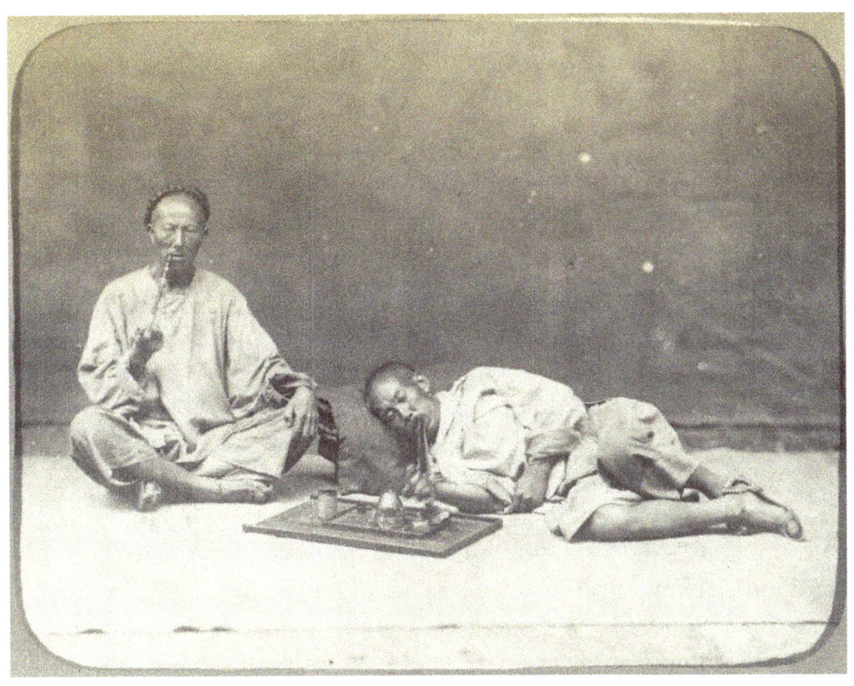

Opium Smoker by William Thomas Saunders 1867
Robert O. Dougan Collection, Gift of Warner Communications Inc., 1981

Smoking Opium

A recipe for preparing Smoking Opium was published in the British Pharmacopoeia in the early 1800s. Basically, it said to dissolve the Opium in water for 24 hours and then express the liquid. Reduce it back to a putty and, again, dissolve it in water. Express the liquor again, reduce, and then repeat the process a third time. For the most part, this process was done to filter out as much non-alkaloid content as possible. When done correctly, one would end up with half the weight, yet twice the potency, that they began with.

For Opium that was made to be smoked, a traditionalist might roll it into the leaves of the Papaver Somniferum. This was the ancient method of storage, and it gives the process an old-world feeling.

When the time comes for consumption, the almost chocolate-colored pea-sized balls are unwrapped and heated until they expand and turn a golden color. It is then stretched and re-balled, heating again to a golden brown. The mass is then placed into an Opium pipe which, in the 18th century, was usually about a foot-long and 2-inch-wide wooden or bamboo tube, with a bowl about two-thirds of the way down. The user draws the smoke in slowly while the flame kisses the heated ball that had been poked into the bowl.

As much as smoking things can be fun, I prefer to eat most of the psychoactive substances I ingest, whenever possible. The effects last longer and are more pronounced. Poppy straw extract, while potent when eaten, is not strong enough to smoke. The amount it would take to feel the high would be hard to consume in one smoking session. Opium smoke is harsh on the throat and the smoking of anything is dangerous to your health. If you plan to smoke Opium, a water bong can help smooth out the harshness of the smoke. If it can be eaten, I eat it. If one wants a quicker method of ingestion, one can make a potion and drink it. Be it Laudanum or poppy tea, the effects mimic that of eating Opium, the only difference being the dosage.

Laudanum

While countless Opium potion recipes were passed down throughout the centuries, perhaps even millennia, the first known Opium elixir was created by Alchemists in the time of the Byzantine, or Eastern Roman, Empire. Potentially the first written formula, the recipe was lost when the Ottomans conquered Constantinople. While we will never know exactly what that tonic consisted of, one thing can be sure. It was mostly Opium.

The first medicine known by the name Laudanum was created by a Swiss-German Alchemist named Paracelsus. He wandered Europe in search of a universal knowledge that was not found in books. While the man had many great thoughts, and many that may be considered quite strange, his belief that the entire universe is one coherent organism is one I find fascinating. He believed that *God* is an organism consisting of everything, including humans. Imagine our bodies, consisting of many different cells and even life forms. Now imagine we are but cells, or even parts of cells, in the anatomy of the Universe. A brilliant thinker, Paracelsus made his version of Laudanum very differently from what became the traditional recipe. It contained crushed pearls and amber, as well as Opium.

There have been many recipes for Laudanum. According to the London Pharmacopeia (1618), the potion consisted of Opium, saffron, nutmeg, ambergris, castor, and musk. This is interesting because, in the right amounts, nutmeg is a hallucinogenic similar to LSD. Other recipes continued throughout the years, each physician promoting their own recipe for Laudanum. The one thing they all had in common, Opium. By the 1700s, Laudanum came to mean a tincture of Opium in alcohol, the other ingredients fell to the wayside as they were ineffective in adding any medicinal value to the final product.

One recipe I've found to be effective is as follows. In two ounces of 120-proof grain alcohol, 10 grams of Opium that has been dried to the consistency of a putty, yet leaves no residue on your skin, is dissolved. The ball of Opium is dropped into the alcohol and let sit for 24 hours, stirring and poking with a sharp object occasionally to promote dissolution. Once the opium is completely liquified in the alcohol, it's filtered through a coffee filter. The solids are discarded, and the tincture is complete. While dosage is variable depending on the potency of the Opium and the weight of the user, two teaspoons, or about 10ml, is approximately equivalent to a gram and a half of the Opium that was added.

Another recipe calls for the dissolution of dried and powdered Opium in 10 times its weight of alcohol. If your Opium is 10% Morphine, this makes the final product approximately 1% Morphine and very powerful. That means a half teaspoon, or about 2.5ml, of this recipe contains about 30mg of Morphine, which would be a rather strong dose for a grown man. Again, dosages vary based on purity, alkaloid content, tolerance, and body weight. Poppy straw Opium is only approximately 1% to 2% morphine and is not a good source material for making Laudanum.

Injecting Opium - Don't do it

What in God's name have you done?

Stick your arm for some real fun

So, your sickness weighs a ton

And God's name is Smack for some

- Alice in Chains

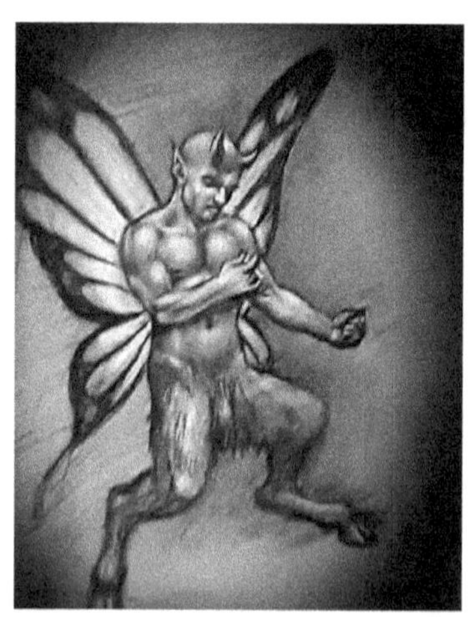

Opium contains fibrous solids and other impurities that make injecting it a very bad idea. There's no high you can get from Opium that you can't get from eating it, drinking it, or smoking it. It's not worth your life to try to speed up the process. If you're someone who feels the need to inject things (Tommy Lee and Nikki Sixx of Motley Crue once injected Jack Daniel's whiskey) Opium is a bad idea and you will probably die.

Opium Potentiators

If you're really trying to maximize an Opium high, there are a couple of things you can do, none of which require a syringe. First, skip a meal. Opiates have a more pronounced effect if they have first crack at your bloodstream. However, if taken on an empty stomach, the nausea is more pronounced.

Grapefruit juice, among other food sources, blocks an enzyme (CYP3A4) from helping your body to metabolize opiates (and other medicines) in the liver. This leads to more opiates in the blood and a longer duration of its effects. Studies show that a glass of grapefruit juice can increase the peak blood concentration of opiates by 1.5-fold. This means that each milligram of Morphine, or whichever alkaloid you prefer, has the effect of one and a half milligrams. That's a pretty cheap way to make 2 grams of Opium deliver 3 grams worth of euphoria. At the same time, the half-life is also increased by almost as much, making it last a bit longer. Instead of 4 to 6 hours, you get 5 to 7.5 hours.

Take it easy. A 51-year-old man was on a methadone program intended to save him from withdrawal symptoms. Instead of getting high on other opiates, he was given 90 milligrams of methadone every day to keep him from going into withdrawal. In an attempt to get high without increasing his dose, or supplementing with other opiates, he drank 2 cups of grapefruit juice a day for 3 days.[11] He was found unresponsive with abnormally slow breathing, pinpoint pupils, and not enough oxygen reaching his body tissues. He had overdosed on his normal daily regimen because of the effects of the grapefruit juice. The only reason that he lived that day was because paramedics found him in time and gave him naloxone (Narcan).

Warning - Drug Synergy

Other substances may enhance and/or transform the experience

The warning on opioids is printed on the label as follows.

Caution; Opioid. Risk of Overdose and Addiction. Ask your healthcare professional if you should have Naloxone on hand in case of overdose. May cause drowsiness. Alcohol and marijuana

may intensify this effect. Use care when operating a vehicle, vessel (e.g., boat) or machinery.

Anyone who has the vast experience with substances that I do knows that this "warning" tells the user that booze and weed will make the effects better. The problem with that is that a lot of overdoses are caused by mixing opioids with alcohol, and marijuana helps quiet the nausea that is the body's natural defense of overdose by vomiting. Opium is its own alkaloid cocktail. It really doesn't need any help. That said, 5mg of THC can complement a cup of Opium tea in a way that transforms the experience from a simple euphoria and body high into a semi-psychedelic mind and body high. Instead of simply feeling elated with a warm, fuzzy sensation throughout, Cannabis adds the thought pattern changes that accompany a good weed buzz.

While alcohol can intensify Opium's fuzzy body high, it only does so until a quantity of alcohol is reached that takes over the experience, dulling the sensation to the point that one only feels the alcohol as if the Opium has worn off. It's as if they merge into a new and unique experience, when the levels are correct, until one eventually submits as the other takes full control. This has the added danger of a drunk person wanting to feel more of the Opium high, thus taking too much, resulting in overdose. I sometimes find that a light dose of Opium, one that would barely be felt on a normal night of even minor alcohol consumption, can be unusually strong when experienced alone.

Another thing to note when mixing intoxicants is as follows: Often, whichever alkaloid hits the brain first wins. By this, I mean that whatever intoxicant you use first can rule the experience. If you smoke some Cannabis and then drink a few beers, you are mostly stoned. The alcohol helps take the edge off of the weed, but the weed is the ruling high until it wears off and gives way to the beers. If you reverse the procedure and get a good alcohol buzz going, then smoke a joint, the odds are the alcohol will hit you like a ton of bricks and you'll be shitfaced drunk. This scenario applies to many different intoxicants, including Opium. If you take Opium before THC, the THC is felt on a lesser scale than if you were to ingest the THC prior to taking Opium. Opium before alcohol has the same result while Opium after a few cocktails can be a waste of time or worse, fatal.

CHAPTER 10
OPIUM AND THE LAW

Legal Status of Opium in the United States
First Opium Laws

Legal Status of Opium in the United States

Many anti-drug laws are mostly the residual effects of Racism. Others were brought upon the world by the self-righteous and religious, often one and the same, who wish to impose their morality on the world. Opium laws, as well as most *anti-drug* laws, are the bastard children of these two corrupt intents. They served both purposes by vilifying the Chinese culture while blaming it for the actions of those they considered their own. The immoral behaviors, such as sexual promiscuity and partying to ungodly hours, were erroneously said to be caused by the practice of smoking Opium.

Many immigrants flocked to California during the Gold Rush of 1849. Among them, the Chinese brought with them their love for smoking Opium. It wasn't long before many Americans joined in the fun. Opium lowered inhibitions and users began to disregard the moral opinions of polite society, even more than usual. To keep the masses in line, the first anti-Opium law in the United States was enacted in San Francisco in 1875. After 5500 years of recorded use (which would be more but for the fact that that's as far back as written language goes), the local government concluded that the smoking of Opium encouraged young men of respectable families to become morally corrupt, and women to become prostitutes. Meanwhile, you could purchase a syringe and a bit of Cocaine from the Sears & Roebuck catalog of the 1890s for a dollar fifty.

The new law banned smoking Opium in Chinese Opium dens. It did not ban Opium. White Americans were not prohibited from purchasing and partaking in Laudanum which, as we know, is Opium dissolved in alcohol. The rich still smoked Opium and drank Laudanum in the privacy of their own homes, going as far as having parties dedicated to the practice. It was only the lower classes, mostly Chinese immigrants, who suffered at the hands of this corrupt system, their way of life being forced underground as Opium smokers became the scourge of society, much like the illicit drug users of today.

In 1906, Theodore Roosevelt enacted the Pure Food and Drug Act, requiring *dangerous and addictive* ingredients to appear on product labels. Opium was still not quite illegal. Food and drug manufacturers just couldn't slip it into tonics without telling anyone. Companies could still put alcohol, Morphine, Opium, Cannabis, heroin, caffeine, and other drugs into their concoctions, which were available over the counter without a prescription, they just couldn't hide the fact that these substances were included, or lacking, in their potions. It was as much about getting all the drugs you paid for as it was about the manufacturer not slipping in some dope, undenounced to the buyer.

In 1909 the Feds followed San Francisco in their anti-Chinese legislation, the Smoking Opium Exclusion Act. Once again, it didn't outlaw Opium. Just the smoking of it for non-medicinal purposes. This was the very first federal law to ban the non-medicinal use of a substance, although many states had already banned alcohol. Let that sink in for a second. Alcohol was illegal before any *drugs* had ever met that fate. It was still perfectly all right for any American citizen who stubbed their toe to walk into a store and pick up some Opium, a little Cocaine, some Cannabis, and a bit of heroin, but if someone were caught in a Chinese neighborhood with a hop in the bowl of a pipe, they would be arrested. Now, the entire country could be done with those pesky slant-eyed immigrants.

Half a decade later, the Harrison Narcotics Tax Act was passed in 1914. As scary as it sounds, the word narcotic having become a dirty word in our society, it still didn't make dope and coke illegal. It only required sellers of Opium and Cocaine to get a license. The act was originally passed as a way to regulate the trade of these popular substances in order for the government to get its slice of the pie. They didn't yet want to ban these *drugs*. Like the Mafia, they just wanted to get their share of the profits. Throughout History, anti-drug laws usually served as a way for the powers that be to keep the poor in line and to collect their cut of the action. It has always been, and still is, legal to sell drugs. That is, as long as you pay your tribute to the bosses.

In 1919 the world of Prohibition began. The Prohibition of Liquor, which banned alcohol consumption and possession, was ratified that year. Next, the Jones-Miller Act of 1922 banned non-medicinal use of Cocaine and Opium. Then came the Anti-Heroin Act of 1924, which banned the importation and possession of Opium for the purpose of synthesizing heroin. The Marihuana Tax Act of 1937 made it illegal to possess Cannabis without obtaining a tax stamp, remaining in effect until psychoactive drug revolutionary Timothy Leary beat the act in court, using the argument that one would have to self-incriminate in order to obtain the tax stamp, thus violating their Fifth Amendment rights under the Constitution of the United States. These laws ushered in a sad time in American history in which the rulers of society decided that feeling any kind of buzz was morally corrupt.

It wasn't until just over 50 years ago, with the passing of the Controlled Substance Act of 1970, that certain medications became truly illegal for recreational use and others illegal for any use. Lawmakers placed all the substances that they thought needed to be controlled into different categories or Schedules, the first of which was reserved for substances that were deemed not safe for use, even under medical supervision. Schedules 2 through 5 were for dangerous drugs that could be used as prescribed by a doctor. Each was considered to have a different level of physical and mental addiction, Schedule 1 being the worst and 5 being the least harmful.

To give you a sense of the lack of knowledge that these lawmakers had, Cocaine, PCP, Opium, and Crystal Meth are Schedule 2 drugs, meaning they have a high potential for abuse and addiction, yet are currently acceptable for medicinal use. Meanwhile, Marijuana is still, as of this writing, on Schedule 1, which states that it has a high potential for abuse, has no acceptable medical use, and that there is a lack of accepted safety for use, even under medical supervision. This flaw in legislation can lead the public to think that smoking pot is worse than doing Cocaine or Heroin. We tell our youth that weed is on the list of the top worst drugs in the world, while Coke and Fentanyl are a close second. Then when they try a little Cannabis and find that it's not that big a deal, why wouldn't they think that the number two drugs are even less harmful? Misinformation is deadly, even when the intention may be that of caution. Good intentions pave the way to hell.

Medicinal substances, and especially the plants they come from, need to be recategorized into more sensible classifications, and safer alternatives to street drugs need to be readily available to those in need. Heroin was made by Bayer, the same dudes that make aspirin, as a *safe alternative* to Morphine that is not addictive. It wasn't long before they figured out that what they were promoting was a load of shit. No one can claim that Opium is more dangerous than her pharmaceutical bastard children. Millennia of use never saw the epidemic that came after alkaloid extraction became commonplace in the last 200 years.

While Americans wouldn't stand for prohibition of their precious alcohol, the first anti-drug law that they repealed, the rest of us were forced to suffer the prohibition of safer alternatives to the bottle. My parents were alcoholics, as were their parents before them, and so on. The only way I was able to escape addiction to both hard drugs and alcohol was with the controlled use of Opium, Cannabis, Mushrooms, Kratom, and other psychoactive substances that helped me forge through the constant alcohol cravings gnawing on my brain. The only thing that quieted the urge was substitution with substances that required less frequent administration. Now I can enjoy a couple of beers, a few milligrams of THC, and the rare but occasional boost of happiness and well-being that comes with Opium.

CHAPTER 11
FINAL THOUGHTS

Everyone I Love is Dead

Everyone I Love is Dead

The war on drugs has many casualties. Most of the characters in my story are gone, fallen while chasing what they believed to be the cure for what ailed them, or the next level of the party. There's a theory I have that better education on how these substances work in their natural state may have led to a different outcome. There is also the possibility that they may have never found the antidote for the ails they were trying to treat and still may have gone to their ends searching, regardless of the substances and information available. Either way, anti-drug laws banning botanical solutions only serve to force these patients underground, into the dark and lonely world of addiction and street poisons that lead only to incarceration and, eventually, death.

Final Thoughts

Papaver Somniferum has inspired mankind and his ancestors for at least 30,000 years. As soon as we learned to scribe legible symbols on clay, we wrote of her power and beauty, a tradition that has never faltered. She is the inspiration for the greatest art to adorn the world's museums and the catalyst for the greatest literature ever composed. From monsters and madmen to poetry and Christmas miracles, our favorite tales began under her influence. Wars have been waged in her name and peace brought about by her euphoria. Rulers have found empathy in her wisdom. She is sympathy and love.

The Opium poppy is the mother of modern medicine, and it would not exist without her. Our symbiosis with her, and all of nature's gifts, is no coincidence. We are meant to be together. Whether a divine gift, a symbiotic relationship, or just an accident of evolution, these flowers are our birthright. No entity can deny us that which is provided by our planet itself. Our descendants will look back at the period of illegal plants as archaic and cruel. Expanding consciousness has been a part of our evolution as a species and is quite possibly the reason for our enlightenment to begin with.

Yet, without great respect for Opium's powerful medicine, we can become entwined in a hellish relationship that ends in suffering and death. Much care should be taken to not become dependent on any psychoactive substance. They are tools, not toys for us to play with. Education should take the place of laws that keep us from them, and guidance should be provided that helps the world understand the dangers and benefits that they bring. Rather than hiding the blade, one should be taught of its use and its potential risks, as hiding the blade only makes it more dangerous when it is eventually found. The same holds true for these medicines.

She is an aphrodisiac and mimics the chemical structure of love itself. She makes the same analgesic chemicals that our own bodies make, yet hers work in a way that ours cannot. She is the one and only plant that does this. And why? The only logical conclusion is that we were meant to be together, be the reason scientific or supernatural. Great men and women have changed the world for her, and because of her. Science has advanced to unprecedented heights due to her presence. After a relationship that has lasted tens of thousands of years, how can we be expected to break it off? She is our greatest pleasure and our deepest pain. None can tally the lives destroyed or the miracles forged for the love of Opium.

THE END

1. ^ Trancas B, Borja Santos N, Patrício LD. O uso do ópio na sociedade romana e a dependência do Princeps Marco Aurélio [The use of opium in Roman society and the dependence of Princeps Marcus Aurelius]. Acta Med Port. 2008 Nov-Dec;21(6):581-90. Portuguese. Epub 2009 Mar 24. PMID: 19331792.

2. ^ Nencini P. The rules of drug taking: wine and poppy derivatives in the Ancient World. VIII. Lack of evidence of opium addiction. Subst Use Misuse. 1997 Sep;32(11):1581-6. doi: 10.3109/10826089709055880. PMID: 9336867.

3. ^ https://www.cnn.com/2010/WORLD/europe/06/30/cleopatra.suicide/index.html

4. ^ *Edgar Allan Poe to Annie L. Richmond — November 16, 1848 (LTR-286)*

5. ^ The Life of Percy Bysshe Shelley, Volume 2 1886 By Edward Dowden p.554

6. ^ The Diary of Dr John William Polidori, 1816

7. ^Neuron VOLUME 98, ISSUE 5, P963-976.E5, JUNE 06, 2018 - A Genetically Encoded Biosensor Reveals Location Bias of Opioid Drug Action - Miriam Stoeber, Damien Jullié, Braden T. Lobingier, Toon Laeremans, Jan Steyaert, Peter W. Schiller, Aashish Manglik, Mark von Zastrow

8. ^ Kumar P, Osahon OW, Sekhar RV. GlyNAC (Glycine and N-Acetylcysteine) Supplementation in Mice Increases Length of Life by Correcting Glutathione Deficiency, Oxidative Stress, Mitochondrial Dysfunction, Abnormalities in Mitophagy and Nutrient Sensing, and Genomic Damage. Nutrients. 2022; 14(5):1114. https://doi.org/10.3390/nu14051114

9. ^ https://www.vice.com/en/article/9bdymy/hamiltons-pharmacopeia-804-v16n4

10. ^ Herbal Aphrodisiacs – Mary Jane Superweed – 1983 - Stone Kingdome Syndicate

11. ^ Ershad M, Cruz MD, Mostafa A, Mckeever R, Vearrier D, Greenberg MI. Opioid Toxidrome Following Grapefruit Juice Consumption in the Setting of Methadone Maintenance. J Addict Med. 2020 Mar/Apr;14(2):172-174. doi: 10.1097/ADM.0000000000000535. PMID: 31206401.

ACKNOWLEDGMENTS

When writing about something that takes hold of your soul, it is easy to be swept away in the process. Long nights and weekends disappear as if no time has elapsed. This would never have been possible if not for my girls. To the spider that crawled into my heart all those years ago and changed the way I see, to the moon that came after to light my darkest hour, and to the evil sorceress that placed them in my arms after a spell of enchantment, I thank you for the continued support and patience as I embark on these journeys. Through you, I am me.

I would have been lost without my publisher, SVDC InDUSTries, and the amazing crew that made this book possible. To my mentors, John, Terence, Anthony, and William, your inspiration shaped my soul in a way that this version of myself couldn't exist without. Because of the four of you, empty people never interfere with my mind. I'd like also to thank my agent, my confidant, and my best friend. Without you, Bill, nothing feels possible. Andy, the greatest artistic mind of a lifetime, thanks for your help and friendship for the last 40 years.

Lest I ever forget, I'd like to thank the Universe for guiding me on a path of my own creation, always taking the time to let me know that [you] are there, ushering me towards my best possible future. I am forever in awe of your majesty, and forever grateful for the second chance you offered. The best is yet to come.

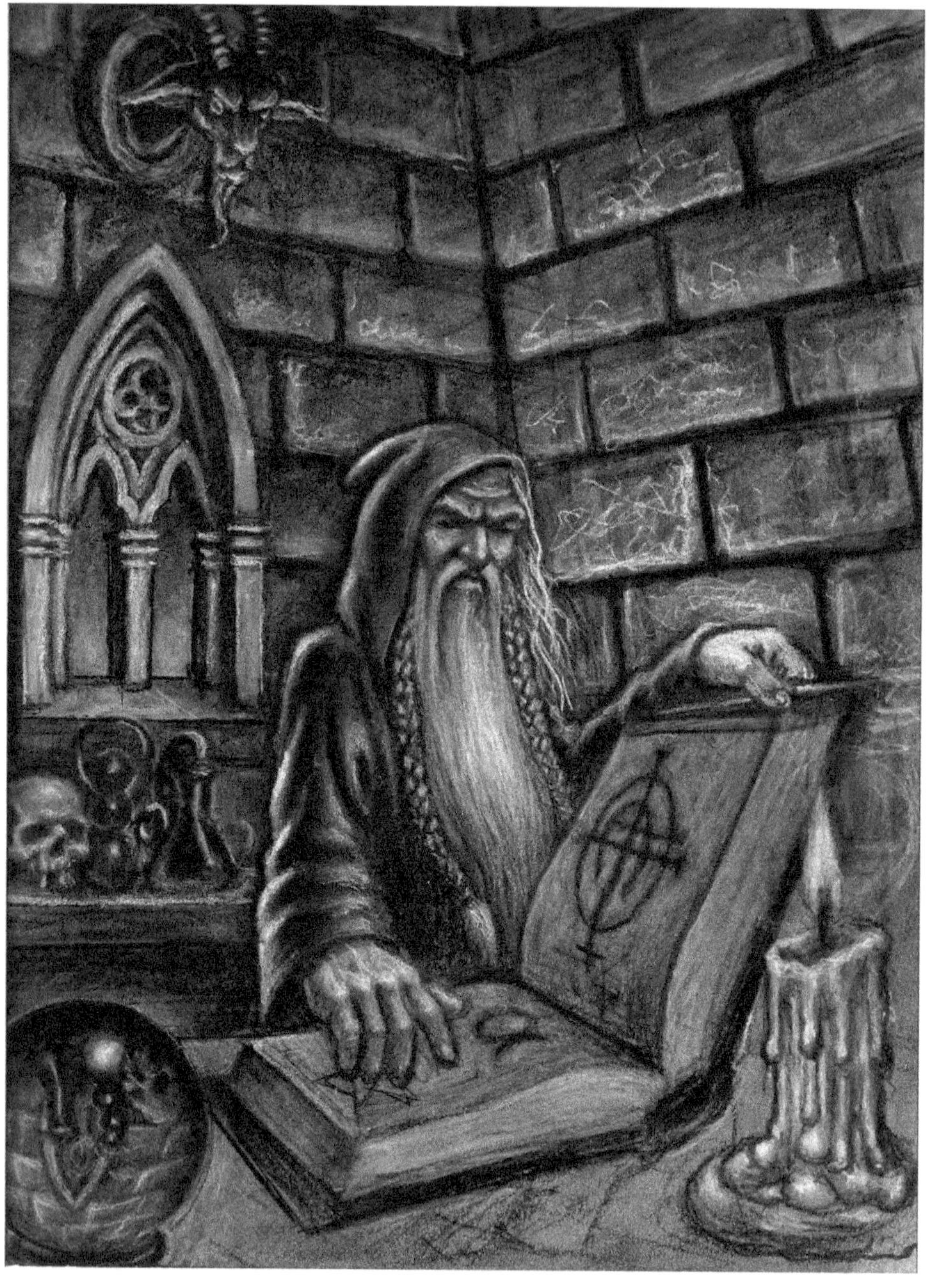

ABOUT THE AUTHOR

W. E. Simmons is an ethnobotanist and researcher from Spring Valley, New York. His introduction to psychedelic substances in the mid-1980s inspired his fascination with their potential for relieving alcohol and substance use disorders. He has spent more than 30 years researching the effects of psychedelics and other mind-altering substances, specifically in the context of addiction recovery. After moving to California in 2002, Simmons dedicated himself to developing a revolutionary method of recovery. With the help of the latest science and a network of recovering addicts, he carefully honed his work into the first truly unique guide to recovery from addiction (and many other conditions of the mind) in almost a century, one that has been successfully used by W. and countless others to finally overcome their struggles. The California Sober method of recovery. In addition to ethnobotany and mind-altering substances, Simmons also authors works in philosophy and fiction. He is an addiction specialist, a medicinal botanist, an experienced psychonaut, and freedom fighter in the War on Drugs.